Contents

Contributors

This book reflects a collaborative effort of the following authors:

Richard W. Albin, Ph.D.
Division of Special Education and
 Rehabilitation
Room 135, College of Education
University of Oregon
Eugene, OR 97403

Jacki Anderson, Ph.D.
California State University at Hayward
Hayward, CA 94542

Felix F. Billingsley, Ph.D.
Area of Special Education, DQ-12
College of Education
University of Washington
Seattle, WA 98195

Edward G. Carr, Ph.D.
Department of Psychology
State University of New York
 at Stony Brook
and
Suffolk Child Development Center
Stony Brook, NY 11794

Glen Dunlap, Ph.D.
Autism Training Center
Marshall University
Huntington, WV 25701

Judith E. Favell, Ph.D.
Psychology Department
Western Carolina Center
300 Enola Road
Morganton, NC 28655

Susan A. Fowler, Ph.D.
Bureau of Child Research
University of Kansas
Lawrence, KS 66045

Kathy Gee, M.A.
Department of Special Education
612 Font Boulevard
San Francisco State University
San Francisco, CA 94132

Lori Goetz, Ph.D.
Department of Special Education
612 Font Boulevard
San Francisco State University
San Francisco, CA 94132

Robert H. Horner, Ph.D.
Division of Special Education and
 Rehabilitation
Room 135, College of Education
University of Oregon
Eugene, OR 97403

Pam Hunt, M.A.
Department of Special Education
612 Font Boulevard
San Francisco State University
San Francisco, CA 94132

Lynn Kern Koegel, M.A.
Carpinteria Unified School District
Carpinteria, CA 93013

Robert L. Koegel, Ph.D.
University of California,
    Santa Barbara
Speech & Hearing Center
Santa Barbara, CA 93106

Pamela G. Osnes, M.A.
Florida Mental Health Institute
University of South Florida
13301 Bruce B. Downs Boulevard
Tampa, FL 33612

Anthony J. Plienis, Ph.D.
Department of Psychiatry
Marshall University School of Medicine
Huntington, WV 25701

Dennis H. Reid, Ph.D.
Psychology Department
Western Carolina Center
300 Enola Road
Morganton, NC 28655

Wayne Sailor, Ph.D.
Department of Special Education
612 Font Boulevard
San Francisco State University
San Francisco, CA 94132

Laura Schreibman, Ph.D.
University of California, San Diego
Department of Psychology, C-009
LaJolla, CA 92093

Trevor F. Stokes, Ph.D.
Florida Mental Health Institute
University of South Florida
13301 Bruce B. Downs Boulevard
Tampa, FL 33612

Acknowledgments ⎯⎯⎯⎯⎯⎯⎯⎯

Early drafts of book chapters were presented by the authors at a September, 1986, conference on generalization and maintenance entitled "Lifestyle Changes for Persons with Autism and Severe Handicaps." Held at Marshall University at Huntington, West Virginia, the conference provided an opportunity for the authors to share their recent conceptualizations and to integrate their work with other findings and perspectives. We are grateful to the administration of Marshall University and to Marshall's College of Education and Autism Training Center for the support and co-sponsorship of the conference.

Generalization
and Maintenance

Introduction

Effective education and behavioral intervention should change the way people live their lives. Throughout this book, we emphasize the point that instructional gains should create practical opportunities and not function as if they were so many merit badges. Hard won changes in behavior should be functional across the full range of situations encountered in school, work, and community settings. In addition, these behavior changes should be maintained for months and years. Currently, we have a powerful technology for teaching adaptive skills and decreasing excess behaviors. This technology will have life-style significance, however, only when it is paired with an applied technology for generalization and maintenance. The purpose of this book is to describe the status of the generalization and maintenance technology needed to translate instructional gains into life-style changes.

The book emphasizes work with students who have been labeled developmentally disabled, mentally retarded, and autistic. These students are some of our best teachers about what does and does not work, and they stand to benefit most from a functional technology of generalization and maintenance. In building the chapters, our objective has been to emphasize three themes: 1) the life-style significance of generalization and maintenance, 2) the empirical foundation for current advances, and 3) practical recommendations for applied procedures. The existing technologies of instruction and behavior management attain full dimension only when combined with procedures for generalizing and maintaining performance gains. Generalization and maintenance connect existing technologies with the values of normalization, integration, and independence.

This book represents many years of intense scholarship by the authors and others in the field. In designing the book, care has been taken to include the behavior therapy and empirical support for the positions espoused in each chapter. Our hope is that this emphasis on empiricism will clarify the recommendations made in each chapter, promote professional debate, and encourage further applied research in this critical area.

The last few years have witnessed a wealth of procedural advances for building generalized gains in community settings. The clinical importance of generalization and maintenance, and recent developments in an applied tech-

1

nology, have provided an impetus for creating this volume. Rather than providing an exhaustive account of all that is occurring, however, the book provides in-depth presentations of those topics that are of greatest applied significance. Chapter 1, by Trevor F. Stokes and Pamela G. Osnes, outlines where the field has been and where it is going with respect to generalization and maintenance. Three "principles" of generalization are provided, and 11 tactics for producing generalized responding are defined. These themes are then illustrated throughout the remaining chapters in the book.

For example, the book explores detailed approaches for building adaptive responses that will generalize and maintain. To illustrate this, Schreibman provides an analysis of the stimulus and consequence variables that affect the role of parents in building generalized skills with students labeled autistic. Koegel and Koegel extend this stimulus control analysis to address pivotal classes of behavior that affect not only targeted responses, but the general "responsivity" of the student to his or her environment, resulting in a "chain reaction" of subsequent development.

If an applied technology of generalization is to have extensive impact it must be useful in a wide range of applied settings. For example, Sailor, Goetz, Anderson, Hunt, and Gee outline the complex nature of community settings and instructional procedures for building generalized skills in those settings. Of particular note in this approach is the emphasis on building instructional trials and consequences within the normal behavioral stream of events occurring in the community. Albin and Horner examined another side of this emphasis on pragmatism by noting that functional generalization requires that the learner both respond in new "appropriate" situations, and *not* respond in new "inappropriate" situations. This is an argument, in essence, for an applied technology that produces generalization with precision. Dunlap and Plienis extend this emphasis further, and present procedures for using "remote contingencies" as an approach for building generalized responding in unsupervised settings. Susan Fowler explores the social context of generalized responding by looking in detail at the multiple roles that peers play in building generalized social skills.

The book also deals with generalization and maintenance of behavior reduction. For example, Favell and Reid provide detailed recommendations for designing interventions that will produce generalized and durable reduction of problem behaviors. In addition, they suggest important strategies for managing staff behavior in settings where behavior reduction is an issue. The recommendations of Favell and Reid are extended by Horner and Billingsley, who provide a theoretical model for viewing undesirable behaviors as "competing" with alternative response patterns. The model provides specific suggestions for assessment and intervention that will lead to durable changes in excess behaviors. This leads directly to the final topic of this book, which shows that a logical implication of the work in the field of applied behavior analysis results in an extremely promising approach for addressing excess behaviors: functional equivalence. Ted Carr brings together a large body of research on functional equivalence and delivers an empirically based analysis of the role that response generalization plays in applied settings. This analysis focuses on the functional effects of responses that produce similar outcomes. The chapter builds from operant theory to specific recommendations for how future behavioral programs should be designed and implemented.

Overall, this book explores and extends existing knowledge related to generalization and maintenance in applied settings. The book provides a window into the research foundation for generalization theory, and outlines a set of practical guides for instruction and behavior management that will have the greatest effect on the life-styles of learners with developmental disabilities, including autism.

Chapter 1

The Developing Applied Technology of Generalization and Maintenance

Trevor F. Stokes and Pamela G. Osnes

There is a consensus that effective applied programs of behavior change should pay special attention to issues of generalization and maintenance. Initially, researchers and clinicians in applied behavior analysis and behavior modification were satisfied with exerting some immediate control over the behaviors of clients. But this success was soon shown to be insufficient for truly meaningful social and developmental changes to occur. Many procedures relevant to the accomplishment of such meaningful changes have been developed, and the principles related to programming generalization have been outlined. The field has progressed, indeed, but there is still some distance to cover before the scientific and clinical pursuits of generalization are well-established operating standards. This chapter characterizes some of the principles, strengths, and shortcomings of the important endeavor of ensuring generalization and maintenance of behavior change.

WHAT IS GENERALIZATION?

There have been many definitions of *generalization*. Traditionally, *stimulus* and *response generalization* have referred, respectively, to the occurrence of behavior under stimulus conditions similar to those of the original training and to

Preparation of this chapter is supported in part by U.S. Department of Education Grant #G008630340 to the authors. The authors also thank the Department of Psychology, University of Western Australia, Perth, for support during the writing of this chapter.

the occurrence of responses similar to the original trained response in the presence of the training stimuli (e.g., Skinner, 1953). These definitions are usually tied to the conditions of stimulus and response variations that may be experimentally linked to the documented generalization. These definitions have much to recommend them, including precision of measurement, experimental demonstration of the functional variables that control generalization, and the pinpointing of basic dimensions of generalization that should be of concern to the researcher and clinician.

The applied literature on generalization has responded to these issues, but not necessarily with the same focus or precision as has been the case with the applied literature on initial behavior change. The outcomes considered important for the practitioner and applied researcher have been clear, though: some transfer of the effects of training to new situations and new behaviors, and over time. After reviewing the extant literature, Stokes and Baer (1977) concluded that, based on the applied research at that time, generalization could be described as "the occurrence of relevant behavior under different, non-training conditions (i.e., across subjects, settings, people, behaviors, and/or time) without the scheduling of the same events in those conditions as had been scheduled in the training conditions" (p. 350).

There has been some controversy about this description. It should be noted, however, that it was not intended to be definitive and was not discussed in such a fashion; instead, it was a pragmatic "notion of generalization." In fact, it was not in the original Stokes and Baer (1977) manuscript submitted for publication, but it was written after a request by the editors. It is clear that the description was topographical rather than functional. That is, some minimal conditions under which generalization may be said to have occurred were described, rather than specifying the functional environmental contingencies that were the cause of the generalization observed. In essence, the "definition" said, if extra effects across various stimulus conditions and responses occur without having been specifically programmed, generalization appears to have occurred. However, if what is desired is an explanation related to behavioral principles and functional contingencies, then a more sophisticated analysis is required. The tactics of generalization programming were similarly presented by Stokes and Baer (1977) as inductive categories, to guide and to challenge, even if they have not all been experimentally analyzed and proven.

For purposes of this chapter's discussion, then, generalization and maintenance involve obtaining widespread change across diverse stimulus conditions, responses, and time without comprehensive programming. As the analyses expand our understanding about the principles of generalization programming, a more precise and/or comprehensive definition may become evident. For now, it is important to note *when* or *where* apparent generalization occurs and to ask

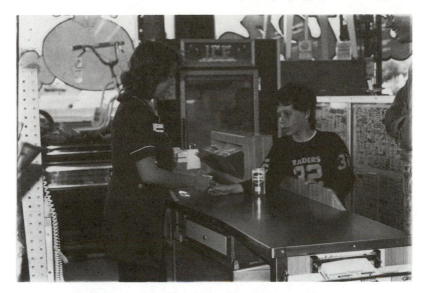

Generalization of shopping skills is tested in nontrained stores.

the critical functional question, *"Why?"* The answer is clearly rooted in the demonstration of functional contingencies in the training and/or generalization situations (Stokes, 1985).

SOME PRINCIPLES OF GENERALIZATION PROGRAMMING

Three general principles of programming for generalization have been discussed by Stokes and Osnes (1986). The first is to *take advantage of natural communities of reinforcement.* In the settings where clients live, there are unprogrammed, naturally occurring contingencies that operate to develop and maintain certain behaviors (e.g., social interaction). To the extent that a program exploits those contingencies for its own gain, effective and efficient behavior change will be accomplished. Widespread and well-maintained behavior change may be observed after initial changes have occurred, provided careful attention is paid to the contingencies operating for that behavior in the "generalization" situation. As some authors have noted (e.g., Baer, 1982), this may not be a "pure" generalization programming tactic, but it is certainly an important guideline when used to maximize the gains of specific training programs.

The second principle, to *train diversely,* runs counter to the frequent notion that the best training is tightly controlled in every respect. It is true that maximum effects may be accomplished in carefully controlled environments without distractions and with presentation of materials and behavior consequences in a precisely managed fashion. However, such effects are often obtained only for those particular circumstances. What may be gained in initial training efficiency may be lost in generalization efficiency. The recommended practice, therefore, would be to maintain the minimum training control necessary for effective change, but to exert as little control over the training conditions as is possible. That is, one should keep the training as loose as possible and incorporate the diversity of natural settings into training as much as possible.

The third principle, to *incorporate functional mediators,* is less mysterious than it may at first appear. This principle recommends that the discriminative stimulus control properties that exist in training may be utilized effectively to facilitate or mediate change elsewhere. Some of those common stimuli are readily observable, such as objects in the physical and social environment that are present in training and generalization circumstances. Some of the functional and effective controlling stimuli are less observable and are carried by the client, such as giving instructions to oneself regarding optimum performance in a particular setting. In all of these cases, the incorporation of functional mediators requires that the relevant discriminative stimuli are present naturally or are artificially introduced into the relevant generalization circumstances.

SOME TACTICS FOR GENERALIZATION PROGRAMMING

Eleven categories of procedures for the successful programming of generalization have been discussed by Stokes and Osnes (1986). These specific tactics deserve incorporation into clinical practice on a regular basis. They also merit thorough experimental analysis to document that they work and why. An outline of each tactic follows.

Teach Relevant Behaviors

Some behaviors are more likely to be reinforced in natural circumstances than are others. For instance, smiling and greeting are probably responded to more consistently and more positively than nose picking. Of course, some attention, whether positive or negative, may follow each of these behaviors. Therefore, if attention is a reinforcer, these behaviors may all have a natural community of reinforcement. The teaching of relevant behaviors has implications in a broader arena as well. If useful and adaptive skills are taught, they are more likely to come into contact with some naturally occurring positive consequences. For example, in Chapter 3 of this volume, Koegel and Koegel describe analyses of environmental conditions that facilitated appropriate behavior of severely handicapped children. The training then focused on "pivotal" behaviors that brought the children into regular extensive contact with the natural (reinforcing) consequences of their environments. Arranging natural consequences for natural behaviors is also discussed by Favell and Reid in Chapter 8. In Chapter 4, Sailor, Goetz, Anderson, Hunt, and Gee describe the development of functional behaviors in relevant community settings.

Modify Environments Supporting Maladaptive Behaviors

If natural reinforcing consequences follow an inappropriate behavior, then that behavior will maintain. For example, when parental attention or peer attention frequently and systematically follows a child's whining and crying, whining and crying will maintain even though there is not a specific program to schedule such events. If the consequences naturally maintaining the inappropriate behavior are discontinued or limited in some fashion, then the inappropriate behavior should decrease in frequency. Of course, a special program itself may be needed to modify the maladaptive environment. In Chapter 2, Schreibman describes how parent training may be used in this manner to modify environments both to decrease inappropriate behaviors and to increase appropriate behaviors. In Chapter 9, Horner and Billingsley describe competing behaviors and environments that may restrict programming for generalization and maintenance.

Recruit Natural Communities of Reinforcement

Some contingencies of reinforcement are not active, yet may be readily activated with minimal prompting. Thus, a person may participate in his or her own program of treatment by actively soliciting the positive feedback and attention that likely will function as positive reinforcers. For example, in social interactions, a moderately frequent cue for positive feedback (e.g., "How am I doing?") is likely to be responded to by others positively, so long as the cue is skillfully given in a timely fashion and the behaviors that precede the cueing prompt are truly deserving of positive reactions.

Use Sufficient Stimulus Exemplars

Materials or situations that vary little in training probably work well to teach performance on those materials in those situations alone. In order to expand the stimulus conditions associated with successful training, a range of stimulus materials and settings can be part of the training. After a sufficient number of stimulus exemplars is incorporated into training, generalization is enhanced. The sufficient number of exemplars necessary varies, but often is small. Albin and Horner, in Chapter 5, discuss strategies of optimal stimulus selection. These authors also demonstrate how negative training exemplars are essential for developing precise responding in generalization contexts.

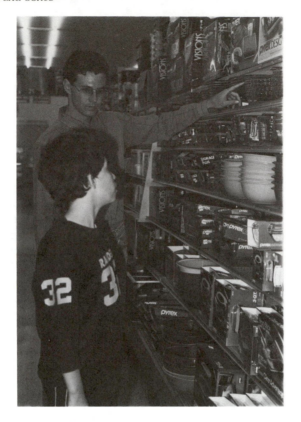

To increase generalization, a sufficient number of stimulus exemplars is needed.

Use Sufficient Response Exemplars

Diversity of response training means that when the performance of multiple related behaviors is the targeted outcome in training, a sufficient number of examples of each behavior should be included in training. For example, developing language repertoires involving correct use of plurals is most efficient using multiple exemplars of plural use in training. The complexity and range of such response classes is discussed by Carr in Chapter 10.

Train Loosely

The principle of diversity of training conditions is well served if the clinician deliberately allows variation to be incorporated into training conditions. The training standard is to ensure that distractions occur sometimes but not always.

An example is when training sometimes occurs in the corner of a room and sometimes in the middle of the room.

Use Indiscriminable Contingencies

Predictability of consequences enables a person to readily discriminate occasions and behaviors that will be followed by positive consequences from those occasions and behaviors that will not. In most training situations, it is desirable that the person comes specifically under the control of the training procedures. In fact, differential reinforcement is typically applied to accomplish such a discrimination. But again, this is a situation where initial gain may become a handicap in the longer term, because effective discrimination may preclude effective generalization. Therefore, in order to enhance generalizability, consequences should be made progressively less discriminable. The sooner this happens in the training sequence, the better. In Chapter 6, Dunlap and Plienis describe examples where unsignaled and delayed consequences were used to maintain appropriate responding in unsupervised settings. These authors point out that generalization was promoted when the contingencies were less discriminable.

Reinforce Unprompted Generalizations

Occasionally, generalization will occur without an apparent reason (or at least one that can be readily discerned at that time). When this happens, an astute trainer who has a commitment to diverse training will seize the opportunity to reinforce the generalization performance, in the same manner as any other target behavior would be reinforced.

Use Common Physical Stimuli

If stimuli are common to both training and generalization settings, and if those physical stimuli assume discriminative functions because they assume a salient role in training, then the presence of the same stimuli in generalization settings may facilitate performance of the behaviors across settings.

Use Common Social Stimuli

Common social stimuli rely upon the discriminative properties of social events to facilitate generalization. Peers, parents, siblings, teachers, and police officers are examples of social stimuli that may become discriminative stimuli for certain behaviors (e.g., polite conversation, aggression). They are likely to function as discriminative stimuli if they have frequently and actively been present or, even more likely, if they have participated in special training in which certain behaviors are reinforced. That stimulus control may then transfer across settings, so that generalization is programmed by systematically introducing the social discriminative stimuli into relevant nontraining environments. Peers are particularly logical targets because they often are naturally present in diverse environments. Fowler, in Chapter 7, describes a systematic program in which peer mediators were very active in the treatment programs of children at school.

Use Self-Mediated Stimuli

To mediate a behavior change is simply to facilitate that change through another stimulus. In the case of a self-mediated stimulus, the mediator is something under the personal control of the target of behavior change. In this way the relevant mediator is carried by an agent of behavior change in order to modify the behavior of the same change agent. Although the process may appear to be straightforward, its implementation may still be risky. The most frequently used mediator is language, produced overtly or covertly (the latter if said only to oneself). The use of self-guiding instructions is one obvious example of the use of a self-produced controlling stimulus. Like other behavior change programs, the problem is that sometimes these manipulations do not work. When they do not, it is most likely that the verbalizations themselves are not truly functional discriminative stimuli or that the mediating verbalizations simply are not produced (see Guevremont, Osnes, & Stokes, 1988). Still, self-management procedures are attracting increasing attention. In Chapter 3, Koegel and Koegel report examples of successful self-monitoring programs used with diverse client populations.

APPLYING THE PRINCIPLES AND TACTICS

To illustrate the application of generalization programming principles and tactics, two cases discussed by Stokes and Osnes (1985) are described here. The first case is that of Robert, a 9-year-old autistic boy who was placed in a residential program because of unmanageable self-abuse in a special school. The residential placement was to continue until Robert's presenting problems had been managed to the extent that he could be reenrolled at the special school. Robert's problems included head-banging, self-stimulation, tantrumming, and noncompliance. A restraining brace was used to control self-abusive hitting. Treatment involved the use of differential positive attention and affection for the absence of self-abuse and the performance of appropriate behaviors incompatible with self-abuse. In addition, Robert's restraints were used as a reinforcer of periods of time without self-abuse and self-stimulation (see Favell, McGimsey, & Jones, 1978).

At the beginning of treatment, one therapist worked alone with Robert. As treatment progressed, the training focus was changed to include multiple staff members in multiple settings (i.e., sufficient stimulus exemplars). In addition, training at the outset included work in a special room and in Robert's typical (natural) settings (e.g., bedroom, bathroom, classroom, gymnasium, cafeteria, hallways, and outside play area [stimulus exemplars]). Various alternative positive behaviors were reinforced. More children were included in close proximity to Robert during activities, and one staff member had to attend to other children as well as Robert (train loosely). The schedule of consequences and the behavior required for the delivery of reinforcers was also systematically altered (indiscriminable contingencies).

In Robert's case, there was considerable generalization within the residential program and in the presence of the staff at other places and times. After a successful course of treatment over 3 months, a teacher from the special school came to the residential program to observe the procedures being implemented and the important progress made by Robert. Shortly thereafter, Robert returned to the special school, and the residential staff provided some follow-up consultation.

Unfortunately, the outcome was less than desirable. Initially, Robert's improvements were maintained for a few weeks after the transfer. There were few instances of self-abuse, and the teachers were able to continue the procedures. Then there was a slight and gradual increase in self-abuse, and the teachers reverted to the use of more "restrictive" procedures to stop him from harming himself. Unfortunately, the program emphasis became less oriented toward the provision of positive consequences for appropriate behavior and became one of reactive and immediate management of self-abuse, which had been shown previously to be ineffective. The influence of the residential program over the procedures was now remote and minimal because a full transition of program responsibility had been accomplished. Residential program personnel restated the successful procedures and urged that they be followed.

The second case is that of Steven, a mildly retarded autistic boy with Tourette syndrome. He engaged in frequent aggression, destruction, and self-abuse. These problems precluded continuation of placement in a school for deaf and blind individuals. Assessment of the functional environment revealed likely contingencies of coercion and escape (see Carr, Newsom, & Binkoff, 1980).

Intervention with Steven involved a differential reinforcement procedure for the performance of behaviors other than self-abuse or self-stimulation. The reinforcing consequences included praise, talk, affectionate touch, edibles, and activities such as listening to music, or loss of access to a preferred ongoing activity if self-abuse occurred. The program also emphasized extinction contingencies for demands and threats and physical guidance following noncompliance, so that Steven could not escape from demands.

One issue at the outset of training included whether to operate the initial training in the regular classroom or in a separate training room. The classroom was preferable but not practical. Therefore, a "classroom" arrangement in the gym was the initial training setting. The program then proceeded quickly from training in the gym to an emphasis on in-classroom training and the incorporation into training of any other setting that would be a regular part of Steven's routine (e.g., cafeteria). Multiple settings and trainers were incorporated as training progressed, in a manner similar to that used with Robert. In addition, variations in appropriate responding were considered acceptable, and more children were added to the responsibility of the staff member working with Steven so that more distractions/stimuli were provided under more natural situations. The intrusiveness of the program was faded as quickly as possible, and behaviors of adaptive value, (e.g., self-help) were systematically taught.

In addition, Steven's teachers and parents came into the residential facility and were taught by the staff to implement Steven's program in a manner consistent with the specialized treatment. After Steven's transfer back to the school for deaf and blind persons, the program staff initially implemented the program in that setting along with the teachers. As the teachers demonstrated clear mastery of the program, the school visitations were decreased in frequency, systematically fading residential program involvement based on the teachers' mastery and continuation of the programming. Steven's behavioral improvements maintained well under these conditions, to the extent that he was later described as a model student.

PRACTICAL ISSUES IN GENERALIZATION PROGRAMMING

Some practical recommendations may be made for the clinician endeavoring to expand his or her own repertoire and develop more sophisticated treatment programs. A practitioner developing skills in behavior analysis and modification is served well by relating successful procedures to the principles of reinforcement, punishment, and extinction. Similarly, the practitioner developing skills that relate to the programming of generalization is well-advised to relate successful procedures to the principles of generalization programming. To do less is to make program development merely technological without understanding the broader context. To be technological is sometimes sufficient, especially in the service of particular clients. However, the victim in the longer term may be the behavior manager, who when presented with a new problem in generalization programming, responds by creating an entirely new set of procedures without building on the past successful applications of principles. It is important that practitioners look for, assess, and analyze commonalities among successful procedures. The commonalities relate to both the procedural similarities and similarities in general operating principles.

A practitioner should also work to generalize his or her own repertoire. Generalization tactics may be applied to the development of the therapist's own repertoire. The practitioner should try to do what works and comes in contact with a natural community of (reinforcing) consequences. He or she should try different techniques so that there is diverse training and success. The practitioner should relate the successful application of procedures to principles, and use the discussion/analysis of those principles as mediators of the planning for generalized changes.

As with any behavior management procedure, the following principle also applies to generalization programming: The better the assessment of functional contingencies and the relevant use of that information, the more likely that treatment procedures will be effective. That is, the practitioner should functionally analyze the occurrence or nonoccurrence of relevant behaviors and the contingencies operating on those behaviors in relevant settings at different times. The intervention techniques should be related to the outcome of the functional analysis. The practitioner should not complete a functional analysis of environmental contingencies and then insert any technique. He or she should work systematically, and the schedule of success will be more favorable.

Again, as with any treatment program, generalization procedures should be written in sufficient detail so that other practitioners can read all relevant information and be able to implement and monitor these procedures effectively. Program managers should be especially careful to monitor the implementation of the generalization programming procedures by practitioners. Direct observation and regular feedback are particularly valuable in this regard.

Generalization programming needs to be built into any serious behavior management program from the beginning of any behavior change procedure. If the focus of attention and effort turns to issues of generalization only after a successful but well-discriminated behavior change, it may be too late. It may be more complicated to work on such programming from the outset, but it is probably more efficient in the long run.

When generalization and maintenance of behaviors are the relevant clinical target, the practitioner should continue to assess the outcome of the procedures throughout their implementation and on a regular basis thereafter. Adjustments should be made in procedures or new procedures implemented when appropriate, as determined by the assessment information. The practitioner should not merely train and hope. Rather, he or she should train and assess, and be flexible in further programming.

The principle of least restrictive intervention should guide both initial behavior change procedures and generalization programming. The more intrusive the procedures, the more they will have to be faded out to more natural procedures. Selection of procedures should also take into account the available personnel and training resources and the payoff to the staff for their consistent efforts.

It should also be noted that there is an ethical obligation, if not a responsibility, to make sure that generalization programming is incorporated into every program that endeavors to make important social and life-style changes for clients.

Developing effective generalization programming strategies is a sophisticated skill that cannot be learned overnight. To demonstrate finesse in generalization programming requires time, practice, and whenever possible, experienced supervision. It may not be easy, but it is possible. The practitioner should learn from mistakes in unsuccessful programs by analyzing them and remembering the errors. One can learn from success by endeavoring to separate effects that are truly the result of the application of good programming principles from those that are due to coincidence, hope, or good luck.

RESEARCH ISSUES IN GENERALIZATION PROGRAMMING

The experimental analysis of the principles and tactics of generalization programming has sometimes lagged behind the development and application of technologies in applied settings. The research literature itself is replete with examples in which generalization and maintenance are well documented, but in which the sophistication of the experimental analyses does not match the promise of the effects observed within the studies. The point to be made here is that when generalization is documented, it should be applauded, but effort should not cease at that time. Whenever possible, there should be an experimental analysis of the variables associated with the occurrence of generalization. Such an analysis will help to refine the tactics and principles of generalization programming.

To increase the understanding of generalization, generalization itself needs to be a major dependent variable, and the generalization programming strategies will likely need to be the independent variables. Advances will not occur unless generalization outcomes are experimentally analyzed. To conduct a treatment study and not analyze the generalization outcomes is the research equivalent of the practical risk involved in the generalization programming method of train and hope. Good luck. Post hoc analyses are simply guesses; they are not demonstrations of causality. The Stokes and Baer (1977) categories are sometimes used to account for the generalization observed, but that is really just appealing to an explanatory fiction. A reasonable fiction perhaps, but it is not proof, at least not in science.

Possibly the future will see a refinement of principles and technologies such that factors conducive to generalization and maintenance may be different. For example, it seems that indiscriminable contingencies and natural communities of reinforcement may be especially important for the occurrence of maintenance. Some techniques such as multiple exemplars also may have particular relevance for stimulus or response generalization. As the research base of understanding of generalization increases, such different factors may become apparent. Or, alternatively, researchers may conclude that generalization is simply an aspect of behavior change accounted for in a straightforward way using the principles of reinforcement, punishment, and extinction. Generalized behavior changes may just be behavior changes with a particular outcome, but not really fundamentally different.

A final point should be made about the evaluation of generalization data. When analyzing research data as a journal reviewer or consumer, it is important to acknowledge that the data of all subjects need not look exactly the same at all times. It has long been clear that no one panacea exists that will reduce all behavior variables to one standard. Variability is often present. To expect all research subjects to always respond to similar procedures in the same way may be requiring too much of the science. The same is true of generalization research. Consistency of data outcome is important, but variations in outcome should also be analyzed to provide information concerning the effects of procedures.

Some variations in research design are also to be expected in research on generalization. It is insufficient to require textbook designs that do not allow for variation. It is also naive to be critical of research merely because it does not fit the established notions of design parameters. Rather, the essential question is what is controlled and how well that control is demonstrated. The field will advance with sophisticated designs judged with flexibility based only on the demonstration of causality.

CONCLUSION

Hope sprang quickly from the initial successful attempts at generalization programming. Train and hope. Sometimes generalization occurred, sometimes it did not. It was a victory to see any at all. Widespread changes were occurring in a cost-efficient manner. Unfortunately, when generalization occurred, it was frequently not clear why. Nor was it clear why generalization did not occur. But at least when it did occur the promise, hope, and aspirations of researchers and clinicians alike were fulfilled.

As might be expected, the hope fulfilled led to rhetoric. Behavior changes could not only be accomplished by differential contingencies, but generalization sometimes was the additional payoff. If it can be done sometimes, there must be a way to do it successfully more frequently. But how? An art was beginning to emerge, a technology of generalization programming tactics that seemed to work. In fact, many fine experimental analyses were built upon astute observations of the art of successful programming for generalized changes. But often it was still not clear why generalization occurred. The prevailing wisdom was that generalization should not be automatically expected, and that the conditions under which it occurred should be experimentally analyzed. Unfortunately, that rhetoric about generalization was maintained more efficiently than the corresponding actual experimental analyses. After all, saying is much easier than doing. It is not easy to complete the comprehensive assessment required of a scientifically sound study of the parameters of generalization. Another source of tension for the researcher is that the research requirements are sometimes far removed from the practical requirements of effective programming. Research tends to be tedious and constraining. Practice is more oriented to prompt outcomes, although it may be frustrating and demanding.

The need for effective procedures is often in natural tension with the extensive requirements of scientific rigor. Yet the field will not advance without the scientific information as its base. The art has come a long way. The science has come a long way. The contributing authors of this book describe some of the best available examples of the analysis of generalization and maintenance and of their programming. But we still have far to go. What have we really accomplished? A great deal, but not enough. We have made an impressive beginning, but there is considerable distance to cover before we have a truly mature art and science of programming generalization and maintenance.

REFERENCES

Baer, D.M. (1982). The role of current pragmatics in the future analysis of generalization technology. In R.B. Stuart (Ed.), *Adherence, compliance, and generalization in behavioral medicine* (pp. 192–212). New York: Brunner/Mazel.

Carr, E.G., Newsom, C.D., & Binkoff, J.A. (1980). Escape as a factor in the aggressive behavior in two retarded children. *Journal of Applied Behavior Analysis, 13,* 101–117.

Guevremont, D.C., Osnes, P.G., & Stokes, T.F. (1988). The functional role of preschoolers' verbalizations in the generalization of self-instructional training. *Journal of Applied Behavior Analysis, 21.*

Favell, J.E., McGimsey, J.F., & Jones, M.L. (1978). The use of physical restraint in the treatment of self-injury and as positive reinforcement. *Journal of Applied Behavior Analysis, 11,* 225–241.

Skinner, B.F. (1953). *Science and human behavior.* New York: MacMillan.

Stokes, T.F. (1985). Contingency management. In A.S. Bellack & M. Herson (Eds.), *Dictionary of behavior therapy techniques* (pp. 74–78). Elmsford, NY: Pergamon.

Stokes, T.F., & Baer, D.M. (1977). An implicit technology of generalization. *Journal of Applied Behavior Analysis, 10,* 349–367.

Stokes, T.F., & Osnes, P.G. (1985). Self-abuse. In M. Hersen & C.G. Last (Eds.), *Behavior therapy casebook* (pp. 342–356). New York: Springer Publishing Co.

Stokes, T.F., & Osnes, P.G. (1986). Programming the generalization of children's social behavior. In P.S. Strain, M. Guralnick, & H. Walker (Eds.), *Children's social behavior: Development, assessment and modification* (pp. 407–443). Orlando, FL: Academic Press.

Chapter 2 _____

Parent Training as a Means of Facilitating Generalization in Autistic Children

Laura Schreibman

As noted throughout this book, the problems in achieving generalization of treatment gains in autistic and other severely handicapped children are legend. These children are extremely difficult to teach, and it is particularly frustrating that newly acquired behaviors typically fail to generalize to settings and people other than those associated with the original training environment. In addition, response generalization is rarely achieved, and the children frequently learn rote responses with minimal variability and with minimal collateral changes in other behaviors. This problem not only presents a severe challenge to normalizing the behavior of these children but also can lead to other problems, such as the lack of neural development discussed by Koegel and Koegel in Chapter 3.

One of the earliest studies specifically addressing issues of generalization of treatment gains in autistic children was conducted by Lovaas, Koegel, Simmons, and Long (1973). This study provided follow-up data on two groups of autistic children who had received 1 year of behavior therapy. One group of children received treatment in an inpatient setting and the parents were not trained to provide the behavioral treatment. Another group of children were

The preparation of this chapter was supported by U.S. Public Health Service Research Grants 39434 and 28210 from the National Institute of Mental Health.

The author is grateful to Debra L. Mills for helpful input.

trained on an outpatient basis and the parents were trained in the principles of behavioral treatment. At follow-up of 1–4 years after termination of treatment, these investigators found that the children who went back to homes where the parents had not been trained, typically lost many of the gains they had achieved in treatment. In contrast, those children whose parents had been trained, maintained their gains and many showed additional improvement. These results added a new importance to parent training for autistic children. Whereas the idea of training the parents seemed like an intuitively good idea (since it involved training multiple exemplars, in a variety of settings, in the natural environment, etc.), it now became apparent that training the parents was essential if one hoped to achieve generalized treatment gains.

There are other advantages to behavioral parent training that make it an attractive mode of providing treatment to these children. First, it allows the parents to participate in the development of their children, something that may have been denied them in the past. Second, knowledge of the cause of the disorder is not required in order to prescribe a treatment. This is particularly important, since historically the parents of autistic children have been implicated in the etiology of the disorder (e.g., Bettelheim, 1967, Kugelmass, 1970). Third, the training is based on principles of learning that are readily taught to nonprofessionals. The literature abounds with reports of parents' successful acquisition of skills and implementation of programs (see Twardosz and Nordquist, 1985, for a review). Fourth, since parents are with their children more than anyone else, training them creates, in effect, an around-the-clock treatment environment. Fifth, parent training allows for the availability of treatment to children who live in rural and other areas where clinics specializing in the treatment of autism are scarce. Parents can travel to such a clinic, receive training, and then return to be the child's treatment provider.

Despite the obvious advantages of parent training and the documentation that such training is necessary for the maintenance of treatment gains, there are problems with training parents that must be addressed before one can consider this treatment modality completely effective. Koegel, Schreibman, Britten, Burke, & O'Neill (1982) compared two modes of providing treatment to autistic children on a number of dependent measures assessing change in parent and child behavior. For one group of families, the children were treated in the clinic and the parents were not trained. For the other group, the treatment was provided solely by the parents, who received behavior modification training. The curriculum for the two groups was the same; only the treatment provider (trained therapist or parent) differed. The results indicated that parent training was superior to direct clinic treatment on a number of dimensions. Compared to the clinic-treatment (untrained) parents, parents who were trained reported a more positive family environment, they spent more time in leisure activities as well as in teaching activities, and they spent less time engaged in caregiving (custodial) activities with their children. In addition, the children whose parents had been trained showed more generalized treatment gains in that their improved behavior was evident in more settings. However, while the generalization of behavior change was superior for the children whose parents had been trained, some serious limitations tempered the enthusiasm for the parent training approach. While the children showed their gains in the presence of their parents, this was not the case when the parents were not present. This was evident both in experimental measures, which assessed appropriate and inappropriate behavior in a structured laboratory setting with parents, therapists, and unfamiliar people, and in the anecdotal reports of the parents, many of whom said that while the child behaved well in their presence, the behavior deteriorated when they were not around. Thus they reported difficulties finding and keeping babysitters, and so forth. It was clear that while parent training led to more generalized behavior change than did clinic treatment, some rather serious problems remained to be solved.

It is apparent that we practitioners need to focus on resolving the generalization difficulties of autistic children before any program, including a parent training program, can be maximally effective. In recognizing this need, investigators over the last several years have directed their attention to understanding more specifically the nature of autistic psychopathology and the particular characteristics that might impede generalization and maintenance of behavior change. The goals of this research are to identify these specific characteristics, develop remedial teaching techniques, and incorporate these improved teaching methods into comprehensive treatment programs. Any procedures thus developed could be incorporated into a parent training package, with the expectation that the problems with generalization previously reported would be reduced or eliminated. Thus, the focus of this chapter is on the nature and the *content* of parent training as opposed to the method of training per se.

Several areas of study hold promise for enhancing generalization of treatment effects. For purposes of clarity, the discussion of generalization is divided into investigations of stimulus variables and consequence variables.

STIMULUS VARIABLES

The study of the relationship of stimulus variables to autistic behavior has had a long and fruitful history. Ever since autism was first identified as a diagnostic entity by Kanner in 1943, the literature has abounded with descriptions of unusual unresponsivity in autistic children. Many of the children have histories of suspected deafness or blindness, as when they fail to respond to their name being called, or fail to notice a significant event in their visual environment such as the comings and goings of people (e.g., Schreibman & Koegel, 1982). There are reports of variations between hypo- and hypersensitivity to sensory events, preoccupation with particular stimuli (e.g., tactile and gustatory), and attenuated pain sensitivity (e.g., Ornitz & Ritvo, 1968, Ritvo & Freeman, 1978). Earlier hypotheses relating to the unusual sensory responsiveness of these children focused on the impact of specific modalities. Thus, Schopler (1965), for example, speculated that autistic children were functioning on a retarded level of development in the normal transition of dependence on near receptors — such as tactile and gustatory cues — to dependence on distance receptors of audition and vision. In an attempt to study the nature of autistic responsivity, Lovaas, Schreibman, Koegel, and Rehm (1971) utilized a discrimination learning paradigm designed to assess the amount of control over behavior exerted by individual components of a complex discriminative stimulus. This paradigm had the advantage of allowing the investigators to relate manipulated aspects of stimulus input directly to behavior. In this study, autistic, retarded, and normal children were trained to press a lever in the presence of a complex stimulus comprised of a visual, an auditory, and a tactile stimulus and to withhold lever presses in its absence. After this discrimination had been established, single-cue test trials were presented in order to assess the control exerted by each component. Results indicated that the autistic children typically had acquired the discrimination on the basis of only one of the components (auditory or visual), while the normal children responded to all three. The retarded children responded at a level between these two extremes such that, on the average, they responded to two of the cues. Subsequent training indicated that the autistic children could respond to each of the components when it was presented in isolation, thus providing evidence that the problem was not one of responding to a particular sensory modality but, rather, of responding to cues in context.

This pattern of responding has been called "stimulus overselectivity" (Lovaas et al., 1971), and subsequent research has addressed establishing the parameters of its effects. After the original study involving three cues in different modalities, Lovaas and Schreibman (1971) conducted essentially the same study, but involving only two simultaneous cues, auditory and visual. The results were the same with the exception that the overselectivity effect was not so pronounced. Subsequently, overselectivity has been found when the simultaneous multiple cues fall within the visual (e.g., Koegel & Wilhelm, 1973; Schreibman, 1975) and the auditory (e.g., Reynolds, Newsom, & Lovaas, 1974; Schreibman, 1975; Schreibman, Kohlenberg, & Britten, 1986) modality. When one considers that most learning requires the control of simultaneous stimulus input (CS-UCS, transfer of stimulus control), it is not surprising that a failure to come under the control of multiple cues would have serious and widespread negative effects on one's ability to learn and to generalize behavior. In a review of overselectivity research, Lovaas, Koegel, and Schreibman (1979) discuss the implications of this pattern of responding for understanding several of the specific behavioral deficits associated with autism. These include the difficulty autistic children have in transferring from prompts (Koegel & Rincover, 1976; Schreibman, 1975), problems in learning from observing the behavior of others (Varni, Lovaas, Koegel, & Everett, 1979), and problems in social behavior (Schreibman & Lovaas, 1973). In a study relating overselectivity specifically to problems in stimulus generalization, Rincover and Koegel (1975) showed how the learned behavior of autistic children came under the control of very specific, idiosyncratic cues in the original training environment. When these cues were not present in an extra-therapy setting, the children no longer performed the behavior. For example, one child was taught to touch his chin when asked to do so. Yet the child would only perform the behavior for the original therapist; when a different therapist requested the behavior, the child did not respond. It was subsequently determined that the child's chin-touching behavior had come under the control of an irrelevant and idiosyncratic hand movement of the original therapist, rather than on the intended verbal discriminative stimulus, "Touch your chin." Since this single cue was not present with the other therapist, the child did not demonstrate the behavior. Obviously, attending and responding to such a limited range of relevant stimulus input can have extremely serious consequences for generalization of behavior.

In attempting to ameliorate the effects of stimulus overselectivity, two different approaches have been successfully implemented. One approach arranges for the design of learning environments that allow the child to learn while being overselective. Such environments arrange stimulus presentations such that relevant cues are not presented simultaneously and the child does not have to attend to more than one cue (e.g., Rincover, 1978; Schreibman, 1975). While effective, this approach has certain limitations in that it is not always feasible to design such programs, and it still involves allowing the child to respond in an abnormal manner. A second, and more promising, approach involves remediating the attentional deficit such that the child's behavior comes under the control of multiple cues. This approach has the advantage of "normalizing" the child's responsiveness, thus allowing him or her to learn in a manner more similar to that of normal children.

The feasibility of teaching autistic children to respond to simultaneous multiple cues was first demonstrated by Koegel and Schreibman (1977). In this study the children were first trained to press a lever in the presence of either an auditory cue (white noise) or a visual cue (red floodlight). After the children had acquired this discrimination, they were then presented with a conditional discrimination in which the S+ was the light plus noise complex and the S−

stimuli were light alone or noise alone. Reinforcement was only available on the complex trials. The results indicated that while the autistic children required many more trials to learn this conditional discrimination than a normal control group, they did in fact learn to respond to multiple cues. These hopeful results suggested that at least for many of the autistic children that demonstrate overselective responding, the potential exists for altering this pattern of attention. One might assume that if the children can be taught to approach new learning situations on the basis of multiple cues, then they should be able to learn in situations requiring response to simultaneous multiple cues, ones that have been particularly problematic in the past. As mentioned earlier, transfer from prompts is one area where these children are noted to have difficulty, presumably because of their overselective attention to the prompt stimulus and subsequent failure to learn about the training stimulus in typical prompt and prompt-fading situations. Could one expect that if these children were trained to respond to multiple cues, they would then be able to transfer from prompts?

To investigate this possibility, Schreibman, Charlop, and Koegel (1982) studied the effects of conditional discrimination (i.e., multiple-cue) training on the subsequent transfer from prompts of autistic children. In a multiple baseline assessment, these children were trained on a difficult visual discrimination. They were provided with an extra-stimulus prompt (trainer pointed with his or her finger to the S+), which was gradually faded. The children failed to transfer from the prompt and did not learn the discrimination. Each of the children was then trained on a series of conditional discriminations involving multiple visual stimuli (e.g., blue bell versus yellow heart versus black clover). That is, the child was trained on one conditional discrimination and, after mastery, was trained on another one, and so on. The training continued with successive conditional discrimination tasks until the child responded initially on the basis of both relevant cues on two consecutive tasks. After the child reached this criterion, he or she was again presented with the original visual discrimination and pointing prompt. As anticipated, after the multiple-cue training, the children then transferred from the prompt and acquired the discrimination.

The results with conditional discrimination training demonstrated that at least some autistic youngsters can alter their breadth of attention and respond in a more normal manner. (There exists the possibility that for some overselective children, the pattern may not be amenable to change via the multiple-cue training described here.) This is an extremely encouraging finding, in that it bodes well for other collateral changes in behavior that might occur if the overselectivity were remediated.

In another study designed to determine the effects of multiple-cue training, Burke and Koegel (in press) used a multiple baseline analysis to compare the effectiveness of two treatment programs on the overselectivity of autistic children and on the collateral effects of each program on the children's social responsiveness and incidental learning. In one program the children then were trained on a series of individual target behaviors (colors, shoe tying, etc.). The second program focused on directly treating overselectivity by teaching successive conditional discriminations (multiple-cue training). Social responsiveness was determined by the ratings of independent observers using a scale designed to assess the child's responsiveness to an adult stranger. Incidental learning was assessed using the "Vocabulary" section of the *Assessment of Children's Language Comprehension* (ACLC) test (Foster, Giddan, & Stark, 1973). This test also contains tasks requiring responses to one, two, three, or four simultaneous verbal cues. When the children were subsequently retested on the ACLC, Burke and Koegel found that the multiple-cue training led to marked increases in the children's responsivity to incidental cues as indicated by their correctly responding to new vocabulary and to other verbal tasks requiring attention to simultaneous multiple cues. This increase was not found after training on individual target behaviors. In addition, when the two interventions were compared on the basis of their effects on the social responsiveness to adult strangers, the results indicated that training on individual target behaviors had no effect on the children's responsiveness. In contrast, after introduction of the multiple-cue training, there was a marked increase in responsiveness.

These studies are encouraging for several reasons. First, as previously mentioned, they suggest that the overrestrictive stimulus control evidenced in the stimulus overselectivity studies is not an unalterable attentional deficit. It is susceptible to remediation. Second, they suggest that remediation of overselectivity leads to positive collateral behavior changes such as the ability to learn from more traditional teaching methods, incidental learning, and social responsiveness. Third, they suggest that the attention of autistic children can be normalized; if this is the case, one can predict that problems in generalization due to overselective attention will be greatly reduced or eliminated.

While most of the foregoing research has involved multiple visual stimuli, this author and colleagues are beginning to address issues of overselective stimulus control within the auditory modality, including its implications for problems in generalization, and remediation via multiple-cue training. Schreibman et al. (1986) assessed the response of echolalic autistic, nonverbal autistic, and normal children to a complex speech stimulus comprised of both intonation and phonetic content components. For example, the discrimination "min min" versus "nur nur!" (where an "!" indicates increased intonation) can be solved on the basis of either content alone, intonation alone, or both cues. The children were taught to press a lever when hearing the S + stimulus and to refrain from lever pressing in the presence of the other stimulus. After the children learned the discrimination, test trials were interspersed to assess which components were controlling the child's responding. As can be seen in Figures 1 and 2, the pattern of responding differed for the three groups. The normal children (Figure

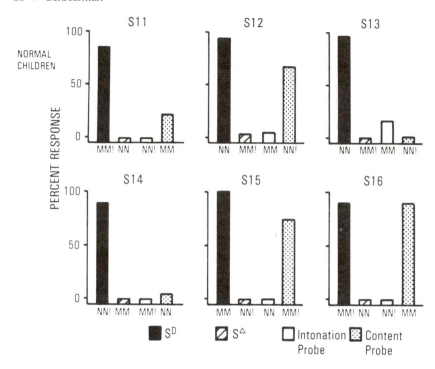

Figure 1. Percent response in normal children to S^D and S^Δ training stimulus complexes and intonation and content probes during testing on discrimination of complex auditory stimuli. MM signifies stimulus "min min" and NN signifies stimulus "nur nur." Exclamation mark indicates raised intonation on second syllable. (Reprinted with permission from Schreibman, L., Kohlenberg, B., & Britten, K.R. [1986]. Differential responding to content and intonation components of a complex auditory stimulus by nonverbal and echolalic autistic children. *Analysis and Intervention in Developmental Disabilities, 6,* 109–125. Copyright 1986, Pergamon Journals, Ltd.)

1) tended to respond to both content and intonation components, as indicated by their response to both content and intonation probes; or if they responded to only one probe, it was the content probe. In contrast, the autistic subjects (Figure 2) tended to respond to only one of the components. Interestingly, the echolalic children tended to respond on the basis of the intonation component, and the nonverbal children on the basis of content. These results are interesting not just because they replicate the overselectivity effect. Unlike the earlier work assessing selective attention to auditory stimuli, this study used speechlike stimuli. The results support anecdotal observations of these children in that echolalic autistic youngsters often demonstrate accurate or even exaggerated intonation when they echo the speech of others—but they may not comprehend any of the meaning. On the other hand, nonverbal autistic youngsters who ac-

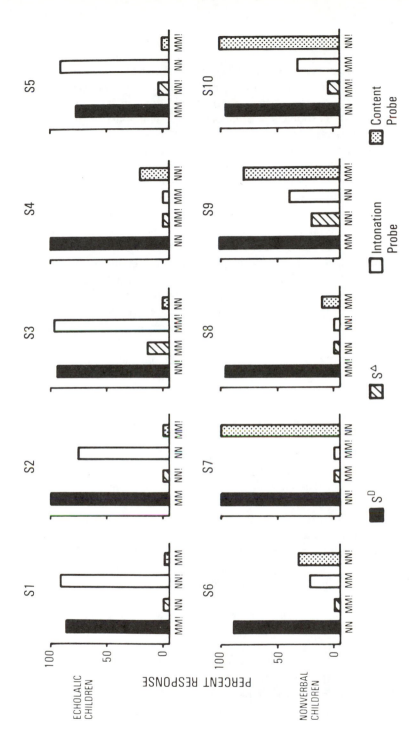

Figure 2.   Plotted in same manner as Figure 1, but with echolalic autistic and nonverbal autistic children. (Reprinted with permission from Schreibman, L., Kohlenberg, B., & Britten, K.R. [1986]. Differential responding to content and intonation components of a complex auditory stimulus by nonverbal and echolalic autistic children. *Analysis and Intervention in Developmental Disabilities, 6,* 109–125. Copyright 1986, Pergamon Journals, Ltd.)

quire language through speech training often sound abnormal when they speak. Thus, while the content may be correct, their speech is often monotonic, and other prosodic features of the speech, such as inflection, pitch, rhythm, and articulation are deficient (Baltaxe & Simmons, 1975; Schreibman et al., 1986; Simmons & Baltaxe, 1975).

If one can generalize from these results, it is apparent that when nonverbal autistic children learn to speak, they attend almost exclusively to content at the expense of intonation and other prosodic features. This could be a function of their language training, in which reinforcement is contingent mainly upon accuracy of content rather than on intonation, pitch, and so forth; also, since these children are likely to respond to only one of the many simultaneous components of language, content would be the one with the most payoff.

This author is now investigating the possibility that conditional discrimination training, such as that already proven effective in the visual modality, can also remediate the overselective pattern of responding described here with speech stimuli (e.g., "min min"); and, if that is the case, whether the children will then respond to multiple components of speech stimuli. In this investigation, autistic children who demonstrate the overselective pattern of responding, as described in the previous study, will receive training on successive conditional discriminations involving multiple prosodic features (e.g., pitch plus inflection, rhythm plus loudness) of speech stimuli. After the children complete this multiple-cue training, they will be reassessed on both the original complex speech stimuli (those to which they previously showed overselectivity) and to a new discrimination, involving complex cues with different prosodic components, to assess further generalization of the training effects. This author anticipates that this multiple-cue training will reduce the pattern of overselecting to one feature of the speech, as found in the original study, and will lead to generalized responsivity to other speech components. It is also hoped that increasing the responsiveness at the receptive level will result in improved prosody of the children's expressive speech.

This focus on stimulus variables has yielded some very fruitful information about how to enhance stimulus and response generalization in autistic individuals. It is both intuitively obvious and empirically demonstrated that by increasing responsiveness to a wider range of environmental stimuli, as in teaching situations, one can achieve generalized changes in behavior.

It remains now for service providers to train parents in how to increase their child's responsiveness to multiple cues. This may be accomplished by teaching the parents how to use multiple-cue training when they present tasks to their children. Thus, parents would emphasize training on simultaneous, rather than individual, concepts. For example, instead of teaching the concepts of color and object separately, the parents could teach the concepts together, as when the child must discriminate between a blue hat (S +), a green hat (S −) and a blue shoe (S −). The acquisition of this discrimination requires response to simultaneous multiple cues.

It should be emphasized that this form of training differs significantly from the way in which parents (and other treatment providers) were instructed in the past. Previously we stressed the importance of minimizing complex stimuli by presenting very simple instructions, using simplified training stimuli, presenting instructions in an invariable manner, and so forth (cf. Schreibman & Koegel, 1981). Perhaps this form of training encouraged response to restricted stimuli in the training situation and impeded generalization. Fortunately, it is now reported that teaching with multiple cues seems to enhance generalization and provides for a more "natural" style of interaction between parent and child (see Chapter 3 by Koegel and Koegel).

CONSEQUENCE VARIABLES

While the study of the relationship between stimulus events and generalization has yielded important information about how to enhance generalization of treatment effects, the study of consequence variables is probably more exten-

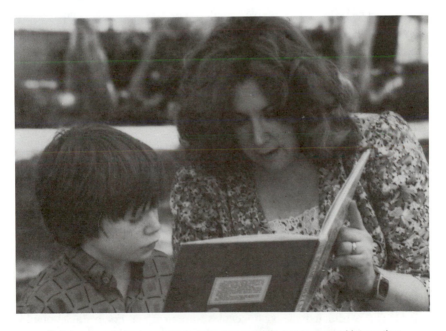

Training parents to use multiple cues can result in a more natural interaction.

sive. Knowledge of the relation of consequent events to the acquisition of operant behavior and of the effects of these events on generalization has proven to be extremely important in the development of effective treatments.

Recent research has focused on two areas where consequence variables seem to hold particular promise for the treatment of autistic children and, importantly, for the maintenance and generalization of behavior change. One of these areas is the effect of consequence variables on the *motivation* of these children to respond in a learning situation. Koegel and Koegel (Chapter 3) describe the teaching of pivotal responses to enhance motivation and the effects of this training on acquisition, maintenance, and generalization. Thus, emphasis on direct response-reinforcer relationships, on reinforcing attempts, on shared control, and on increased success have been demonstrated to increase the children's motivation to respond and their generalization of behavior, as well as enhancing other, collateral, behaviors. The procedures described by Koegel and Koegel in this volume can be easily incorporated into a parent training program and also closely approximate "normal" parent-child interactions.

The other area of recent research relates to the consistency of delivery of the consequences. While this author and others have been diligent in emphasizing to parents the importance of being "consistent" about the application of consequences, it appears that this consistency may in fact inhibit the generalized effects for which we strive. While consistency may be crucial to the accomplishment of the initial behavior change, it can be problematic when the children use this consistency to identify which environments are, and are not, contingent. Thus the children often become masters at discriminating environments, and their behavior changes with changing environments. Anyone working with these children can provide examples of youngsters who behave well when they know contingencies are in effect (e.g., the mother is in the room), only to display inappropriate behavior when it is apparent that contingencies are not in effect (e.g., a stranger is in the room). It is this ability to discriminate environments that impedes generalized effects. One way to make the environments less discriminable is to make the operating contingencies less discriminable; that is, to make them inconsistent.

This author and colleagues have begun to explore two specific arrangements of consequences to make their delivery inconsistent. One is to make the occasion for consequence delivery inconsistent across time and the other is to make the specific consequence inconsistent. This author's pilot work in the first area has sought to investigate the feasibility of applying effective consequences inconsistently so that the child cannot discriminate the occasion for consequence delivery. Under these circumstances one might expect that the child would behave as though the contingencies were in effect. For example, one 14-year-old autistic child known to the author engaged in delayed echolalia of television programs. This behavior worried his parents, because it made him look deviant, and they feared others might react literally to such expressions and try to "take advantage of him." He would not engage in this behavior when his parents, sister, teacher, or therapists were with him, since he knew that these individuals would be contingent in their delivery of verbal punishers for the psychotic speech. However, when none of these individuals was nearby, and a stranger was present, he would almost immediately begin to engage in the bizarre talk. The parents reported that even though they were not near him, they knew when he was doing it because they could see the startled expressions on the faces of those around him. Basically, the youngster would say one word or phrase and if the stranger did not apply a consequence (which would, of course, be the most common occurrence), he would discriminate that this was a noncontingent environment and would continue to talk. This author reasoned that if the discrimination could be made an unreliable one, then this child might suppress his psychotic speech in noncontingent environments. One way to make this discrimination unreliable is to have strangers be contingent some of the time and noncontingent some of the time. Thus, the child would learn that even though this stranger is not contingent now, he or she might be contingent in 10 seconds. Under these conditions, one might expect suppression of the behavior, since the environment could not be identified as completely noncontingent. The author's pilot work in this area suggests that this indeed promises to be an effective procedure for enhancing generalized suppression of inappropriate behavior. These data suggest that once an effective consequence is identified, and used in a consistent and contingent manner to ensure effectiveness, a shift to contingency delivery from 100% of the time to about 33% of the time yields positive results. However, it appears that the inconsistency must be programmed and carefully monitored; it cannot be haphazard. While this procedure awaits validation with additional data, the results so far are encouraging.

While enhanced generalization is an obvious benefit of the application of inconsistent contingent consequences, another positive feature of such consequences is that they contribute to a more "natural" interaction pattern between parent and child. Thus, while parents may try to be consistent, it is often just not possible.

Another strategy under investigation by this author for programming inconsistency in consequence delivery may be appropriate for children for whom effective consequences, applied consistently, lose their effectiveness over time. Thus, while a parent has found a specific consequence (e.g., timeout) to be effective for controlling tantrums, this consequence may subsequently become ineffective. Under these conditions, the parent, or other caregiver, may get discouraged and go back to "old" ways of dealing with the behavior or may keep trying more and more severe controlling consequences. Figure 3 presents some pilot data with one child who engaged in very intense self-stimulation that often escalated to the point of being aggressive and/or self-injurious. As can be seen from the graph, several initially effective consequences lost effectiveness over time. These included such tried-and-true punishers as timeout, having the child put his head down into his lap, having the child hold his arms up and away from his body, and a slap to the thigh. In the experimental condition, all of the previously effective consequences were alternated on a randomized basis such that the child could not predict which of the consequences would be applied to the next instance of self-stimulation. Under these conditions, the behavior dropped to a very low rate and remained under control for 11 months (at which time the child was no longer available to participate in the research). These results are encouraging in that they provide support for a procedure that may have utility in those cases where consequences lose effectiveness. Such procedures may ultimately help to reduce the aversiveness of treatment interventions and the reliance on extreme punishers. There are also data suggesting that simply varying punishers (independent of previous effectiveness) may serve to enhance suppressive effects without using severe punishers (Charlop, Burgio, Iwata, & Ivancic, in press).

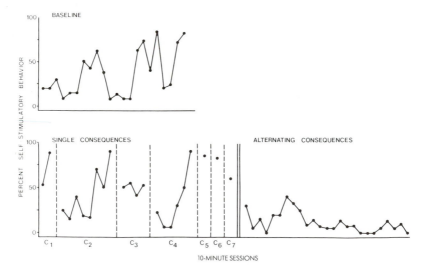

Figure 3. Percent occurrence of self-stimulation in an autistic child during 10-second continuous interval recording. Each data point represents 10-minute session. During baseline, no consequences were applied to the behavior. (C_1 = timeout, C_2 = head in lap, C_3 = arms up, C_4 = slap on thigh, C_5 = turn away with food tray, C_6 = ice pack, C_7 = verbal reprimands.)

SOCIAL VALIDATION ASSESSMENT

Investigators with an applied behavior analytic perspective have employed a variety of measures to allow for the comprehensive and detailed assessment of generalization. These have included thorough evaluation of generalization across settings and other stimulus environments, generalization within and across response classes, and the durability of behavior change over time. It is only through the use of these measures in systematic investigations that researchers have been able to be precise about functional variables meriting study in the quest for techniques to enhance generalization.

Another assessment methodology has now become available to behavior analysts that allows us to ask questions about the broader impact of our treatments. This methodology, known as social validation, seeks to determine the social importance and/or acceptability of treatment targets, procedures, and effects. Using this methodology, it is possible to obtain information on the true generality of treatment effects in terms of the response of significant others in the children's environment to the child's behavior. In this case, significant others also include members of the general public, since it is always hoped that these children will spend more and more of their time in the "normal" environment.

An initial study (Schreibman, Koegel, Mills, & Burke, 1981) was designed to assess whether behavioral changes measured by objective observational measures correlated with behavior changes noted by naive judges in subjective ratings of autistic children at pre- and at posttreatment. Groups of undergraduate students viewed pre- and posttreatment videotape segments of each of several autistic children. The videotaped segments were viewed in a randomized order and the judges were not told that the children were autistic nor that they were receiving treatment. After each viewing the judges filled out a questionnaire containing several Likert-type questions about the extent to which the child engaged in specific behaviors (e.g., repetitive behavior, imitates the speech of others, plays with toys) as well as items on a social distance scale designed to assess how close the judge was willing to be to the child (e.g., "I would be willing to babysit for this child"). There were also global judgment items such as "This child appears abnormal" and "I like this child." As a basis for comparison, the videotaped segments were also scored according to the investigators' objective observational scheme, which scored individual appropriate and inappropriate behaviors during 10-second continuous intervals. The children were divided into two groups based on the authors' objective measures, one group comprising those who showed significant improvement and the other comprising those who did not. In studying the correlations between the children who showed improvement on the objective measures and those for whom the subjective impressions suggested significant improvement, the results were highly significant. In addition, there were significant correlations between individual questionnaire items (e.g., child imitates speech of others) and individual objective scoring (e.g., echolalia). These results not only suggest that the improvements measured by the objective measures were correlated with improvements as seen by naive judges, but also that the specific generalization assessments used in the laboratory were based on the same behaviors used by the raters to make their subjective judgments.

Because of the direct influence of significant others on the life of the child, one could argue that the most significant others in the autistic child's environment are the parents and teachers. In modified replications of the Schreibman et al. (1981) study, these populations were used to provide the subjective impressions (Runco & Schreibman, 1983; Schreibman, Runco, Mills, & Koegel, 1982). Basically, it was found that teachers and parents also noted the changes in the children to a degree consistent with the objective measures, and that the specific behaviors used to make these judgments may be different.

With this kind of generalization technology, it is possible not only to determine the generality of treatment *effects* but also specifics of which behaviors are important to which relevant consumer. Obviously, this information would be quite useful in designing treatment programs to have maximal effectiveness with relevant consumers. An additional way to obtain vital information about what relevant consumers find important is to use social validation methodology to look at the *focus* of treatment. Runco and Schreibman (1987) showed videotapes of autistic children to groups of parents of autistic children and therapists and asked them to rate the importance of various behaviors (e.g., noncooperation, echolalia, self-stimulation) for treatment intervention. As the researchers had anticipated, parents and therapists differed in their perceptions of which behaviors are most important for treatment. For example, parents judged all categories of behavior (e.g., play behaviors, general appearance, verbal behaviors, interactive/noninteractive behaviors) as more important treatment targets than did teachers or therapists. Also, all judges viewed noninteractive behaviors as the most important objective of treatment. Any successful parent training program needs to consider the judgments of parents as important input in decisions on training targets. It should also be noted that parents may not view as important those behaviors known to have generalized effects on future functioning (e.g., certain verbal behaviors), and in these cases it may be vital to educate the parents about these factors so that they can then make a more informed judgment (Runco & Schreibman, 1987).

INCORPORATION OF GENERALIZATION PROCEDURES IN PARENT TRAINING

With the identification of procedures that enhance the probability of achieving generalization, the next step is to incorporate these procedures into an im-

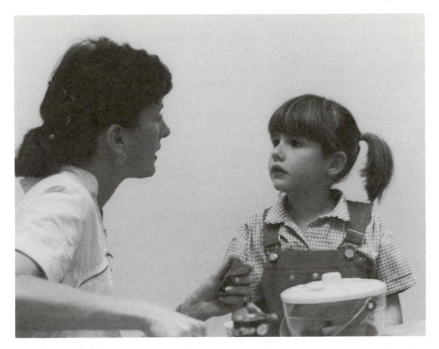

Parents can readily incorporate generalization-enhancing procedures when teaching their children.

proved parent training package. With recent studies addressing these issues with autistic children, researchers may now be ready to take the first steps in this direction. As discussed by Koegel and Koegel in Chapter 3, researchers have uncovered some very promising new leads into ways to increase the motivation of these children. The research presented in the current chapter suggests that a generalized increase in responsivity is possible and, when accomplished, leads to changes in collateral behaviors. In addition, modifications in consequence variables have been identified that may enhance generalization. What is needed now is a field-test of a package containing these procedures and, subsequently, a component analysis to assist in the identification of the most effective and efficient training package.

Responding to the limitations noted by others in the area of research in training parents of autistic children, Laski, Charlop, and Schreibman (in press) implemented a parent training package consisting of several specific generalization-enhancing features. This program was based on the speech training program described by Koegel, O'Dell, and Koegel (1987) and included procedures such as shared control (turn taking), reinforcing attempts to speak, frequent variation of task, and direct response-related reinforcement (e.g., access to toy or activity). Parents of four nonverbal autistic children were instructed in this language training package during a multiple baseline analysis. Treatment effects were assessed in three nontreatment locations, a clinic playroom, a home free-play setting, and a clinic waiting room. Three categories of parent behaviors were measured, including: 1) the frequency with which parents requested that their child perform a nonverbal behavior (e.g., "Bring me the ball"), 2) the frequency with which parents requested that their child respond with a vocalization (e.g., parent prompted the child to answer a question), and 3) the frequency with which parents engaged in general talk with their child. Three categories of child verbal behaviors were measured: 1) imitations of parents' vocalizations, 2) responses that were not direct imitations (e.g., which were answers to questions), and 3) spontaneous vocalizations. The results of this study indicated that during baseline, parents more frequently requested that their children respond nonverbally than verbally. Following the training, all parents increased the frequency with which they modeled appropriate words and phrases for their child to imitate, prompted verbal responses, and required their child to respond verbally. In addition, the parents increased their general talk with their children and also decreased their requests for nonverbal behaviors. Looking at the changes in the children's verbal behavior, the results are especially encouraging. Verbal imitation increased for all children, as did answers to questions and spontaneous speech. These data suggest that parents of autistic children can produce generalized speech gains by incorporating generalization-enhancing procedures as described here. Of significance is that these data also suggest that parent training with these procedures may have the positive effect of changing the way parents verbally interact with their autistic children.

Laski et al. (in press) provide us with an exciting beginning, one that bodes well for an improved parent training package that includes features known to enhance generalization. What remains to be done is a further analysis of such a training package, including procedures known to enhance responsivity in these children. One might predict that such a program might be even more successful than the one used by Laski et al. Further, it is imperative to continue to assess the effects of this training on family variables such as stress-reduction, everyday activities, family environment, and parental satisfaction. Such research is currently underway, and it is predicted that this new parent training program will lead to more positive effects on the family than previously achieved and will result in significantly improved generalization of treatment effects with the children.

REFERENCES

Baltaxe, C.A.M., & Simmons, J.Q. (1975). Language in childhood psychosis: A review. *Journal of Speech and Hearing Disorders, 30,* 439–458.

Bettelheim, B. (1967). *The empty fortress.* New York: Free Press.

Burke, J.C., & Koegel, R.L. (in press). Some generalized effects of multiple-cue training: A longitudinal assessment. *Journal of Experimental Child Psychology.*

Charlop, M.H., Burgio, L.D., Iwata, B.A., & Ivancic, M.T. (in press). Stimulus variation as a means of enhancing punishment effects. *Journal of Applied Behavior Analysis.*

Foster, R., Giddan, J.J., & Stark, J. (1973). *Assessment of Children's Language Comprehension.* Palo Alto, CA: Consulting Psychologists Press, Inc.

Kanner, L. (1943). Autistic disturbances of affective contact. *Nervous Child, 3,* 217–250.

Koegel, R.L., O'Dell, M.C., & Koegel, L.K. (1987). A natural language teaching paradigm for nonverbal autistic children. *Journal of Autism and Developmental Disorders, 17,* 187–200.

Koegel, R.L., & Rincover, A. (1976). Some detrimental effects of using extra stimuli to guide learning in normal and autistic children. *Journal of Abnormal Child Psychology, 4,* 59–71.

Koegel, R.L., & Schreibman, L. (1977). Teaching autistic children to respond to simultaneous multiple cues. *Journal of Experimental Child Psychology, 24,* 299–311.

Koegel, R.L., Schreibman, L., Britten, K.R., Burke, J.C., & O'Neill, R.E. (1982). A comparison of parent training to direct clinic treatment. In R.L Koegel, A. Rincover, & A.L. Egel (Eds.), *Educating and understanding autistic children* (pp. 260–280). San Diego: College-Hill Press.

Koegel, R.L., & Wilhelm, H. (1973). Selective responding to the components of multiple visual cues by autistic children. *Journal of Experimental Child Psychology, 15,* 442–453.

Kugelmass, N.I. (1970). *The autistic child.* Springfield, IL: Charles C Thomas.

Laski, K.E., Charlop, M.H., & Schreibman, L. (in press). Training parents to use the Natural Language Paradigm to increase their autistic children's speech. *Journal of Applied Behavior Analysis.*

Lovaas, O.I., Koegel, R.L., & Schreibman, L. (1979). Stimulus overselectivity and autism: A review of research. *Psychological Bulletin, 86,* 1236–1254.

Lovaas, O.I., Koegel, R.L., Simmons, J.Q., & Long, J.S. (1973). Some generalization and follow-up measures on autistic children in behavior therapy. *Journal of Applied Behavior Analysis, 6,* 131–166.

Lovaas, O.I., & Schreibman, L. (1971). Stimulus overselectivity of autistic children in a two-stimulus situation. *Behaviour Research and Therapy, 9,* 305–310.

Lovaas, O.I., Schreibman, L., Koegel, R.L., & Rehm, R. (1971). Selective responding by autistic children to multiple sensory input. *Journal of Abnormal Psychology, 77,* 211–222.

Ornitz, E.M., & Ritvo, E.R. (1968). Perceptual inconstancy in early infantile autism. *Archives of General Psychiatry, 18,* 76–98.

Reynolds, B.S., Newsom, C.D., & Lovaas, O.I. (1974). Auditory overselectivity in autistic children. *Journal of Abnormal Child Psychology, 2,* 253–263.

Rincover, A. (1978). Variables affecting stimulus-fading and discriminative responding in psychotic children. *Journal of Abnormal Psychology, 87,* 541–553.

Rincover, A., & Koegel, R.L. (1975). Setting generality and stimulus control in autistic children. *Journal of Applied Behavior Analysis, 8,* 235–246.

Ritvo, E.R., & Freeman, B.J. (1978). National Society for Autistic Children definition of the syndrome of autism. *Journal of Autism and Childhood Schizophrenia, 8,* 235–246.

Runco, M.A., & Schreibman, L. (1983). Parental judgments of behavior therapy efficacy with autistic children: A social validation. *Journal of Autism and Developmental Disorders, 13,* 237–248.

Runco, M.A., & Schreibman, L. (1987). Socially validating behavioral objectives in the treatment of autistic children. *Journal of Autism and Developmental Disorders, 17,* 141–147.

Schopler, E. (1965). Early infantile autism and receptor processes. *Archives of General Psychiatry, 13,* 327–335.

Schreibman, L. (1975). Effects of within-stimulus and extra-stimulus prompting on discrimination learning in autistic children. *Journal of Applied Behavior Analysis, 8,* 91–112.

Schreibman, L., Charlop, M.H., & Koegel, R.L. (1982). Teaching autistic children to use extra stimulus prompts. *Journal of Experimental Child Psychology, 33,* 475–491.

Schreibman, L, & Koegel, R.L. (1981). A guideline for planning behavior modification programs for autistic children. In S. Turner, K. Calhoun, & H. Adams (Eds.), *Handbook of clinical behavior therapy* (pp. 500–526). New York: John W. Wiley & Sons.

Schreibman, L., & Koegel, R.L. (1982). Multiple cue responding in autistic children. In J. Steffen & P. Karoly (Eds.), *Advances in child behavioral analysis and therapy, Vol. II: Autism and severe psychopathology* (pp. 81–102). Lexington, MA: D.C. Heath.

Schreibman, L., Koegel, R.L., Mills, J.I., & Burke, J.C. (1981). Social validation of behavior therapy with autistic children. *Behavior Therapy, 12,* 610–624.

Schreibman, L., Kohlenberg, B.S., & Britten, K.R. (1986). Differential responding to content and intonation components of a complex auditory stimulus by nonverbal and echolalic autistic children. *Analysis and Intervention in Developmental Disabilities, 6,* 109–125.

Schreibman, L., & Lovaas, O.I. (1973). Overselective response to social stimuli by autistic children. *Journal of Abnormal Child Psychology, 1,* 152–168.

Schreibman, L., Runco, M.A., Mills, J.I., & Koegel, R.L. (1982). Teachers' judgments of improvements in autistic children in behavior therapy: A social validation. In R.L. Koegel, A. Rincover, & A.L. Egel (Eds.), *Educating and understanding autistic children* (pp. 78–87). San Diego: College-Hill Press.

Simmons, J.Q., & Baltaxe, C. (1975). Language patterns of adolescent autistics. *Journal of Autism and Childhood Schizophrenia, 5,* 333–351.

Twardosz, S., & Nordquist, V.M. (1985). Parent training. In M. Hersen & V.B. Van Hesselt (Eds.), *Behavior therapy with children and adolescents: A clinical approach* (pp. 75–105). New York: John Wiley & Sons.

Varni, J.W., Lovaas, O.I., Koegel, R.L., & Everett, N.L. (1979). An analysis of observational learning in autistic and normal children. *Journal of Abnormal Child Psychology, 7,* 31–43.

Chapter 3

Generalized Responsivity and Pivotal Behaviors

Robert L. Koegel and Lynn Kern Koegel

One of the major characteristics of persons with developmental disabilities, such as autism, is a marked failure to respond to environmental stimuli (Anthony, 1958; Kanner, 1943; Lovaas, Koegel, & Schreibman, 1979; Ornitz, 1974; Schopler, 1965). In contrast to normal children who are characterized by a sheer prevalence of responding to practically anything and everything in their environment, autistic children are typically unresponsive to the majority of environmental stimuli. O'Neill (1987) provided data showing that in comparison to normal children in a playroom setting, autistic children typically responded much less frequently to the stimuli (e.g., toys, furniture, paintings, people) in the room. Second, the autistic children did not shift from one stimulus to another on the occasions when they did respond, but usually perseverated in responding to a single stimulus. Also, they did not respond to complex (multiple-component) stimuli, nor did they combine one stimulus with another, or attempt to relate one stimulus to another (e.g., build things with blocks, or put one object inside another). Finally, they did not survey all of the available stimuli in the room before selecting a preferred stimulus. Of particular concern in this chapter is the implication that such failures to respond to environmental stimuli could seriously impair neurological and behavioral development.

The present discussion focuses on treatment approaches that target responsivity as a pivotal target behavior, and that have the potential to produce

Portions of the research discussed in this chapter were supported by U.S. Public Health Service Research Grants MH28210 and MH39434 from the National Institute of Mental Health, and by the U.S. Department of Education, Special Education Program Contract No. 300-82-0362.

Appreciation is expressed to Robert O'Neill, John C. Burke, and Jean Johnson for their assistance.

widespread developmental improvements in the children's behavior. *Responsivity,* as it relates to this research, is defined as occurring when an individual: 1) makes relatively frequent responses to environmental stimuli, 2) switches responses relatively frequently from one stimulus to another, 3) makes relatively more responses to complex (multiple-component) stimuli than to single stimuli, and 4) makes frequent responses that combine or relate one stimulus to another. The literature reviewed here suggests that the absence of any of these characteristics would be likely to result in a subsequent chain of severely abnormal development because of the consequent sensory deprivation produced by unresponsivity, and because of the reduced opportunities for learning produced by unresponsivity. Two approaches to producing increases in the children's responsivity, with minimal therapist effort, are: 1) targeting the children's motivation to respond to their environment and 2) teaching the children to self-monitor their environmental interactions so that they respond appropriately across multiple environments. Each of these areas is discussed in detail in this chapter, following an overview of the neurological and behavioral reasons related to the importance of focusing on responsivity as a pivotal target behavior.

NEUROLOGICAL IMPLICATIONS OF UNRESPONSIVITY

A wide variety of research in sensory deprivation and in enriched vs. impoverished environments suggests that: 1) neurological development is impaired by a lack of response to environmental stimulation and 2) enriched environments, providing optimal levels of stimulation, appear to improve both normal and abnormal neurological functioning (Greenough, 1984; Greer, Diamond, & Tang, 1982).

Sensory Deprivation as a Result of Unresponsivity

Sensory deprivation is defined as a period of time when an individual experiences an absence of sensory stimulation (cf. R. L. Koegel & Felsenfeld, 1977). *Sensory stimulation,* in turn, is defined as any change in stimulation experienced by an individual. Therefore, sensory deprivation effects are incurred not only when an individual is in an environment with relatively few stimuli but also when the individual fails to respond to existing stimuli. Similarly, when there is relatively little variation or change in responding to those stimuli, sensory deprivation effects are likely to occur. Thus, the absence of variation in intensity, complexity, movement, contrast, pitch, texture, hue, and so forth, can all result in sensory deprivation effects (cf. Fiske & Maddi, 1961; Riesen & Zilbert, 1975). This is important to note in relation to O'Neill's results (described earlier), which show that autistic children have response abnormalities in many such areas. For example, failure either to respond to stimuli or to switch responding from one stimulus to another would both be expected to place the child in a sensory-deprived environment. Further, failing to respond to complex (multiple-component) stimuli would be expected to result in a severe degree of sensory deprivation (Finger & Stein, 1982). That is, the present authors suggest that responses to single-component stimuli are not enough to advance neurological development; and that responses that associate components of complex stimuli are essential for normal development. It may also be important to consider such sensory deprivation and developmental implications in relation to the stimulus overselectivity characteristic in autism, where such children fail to respond to many of the components of complex stimuli (see Schreibman, Chapter 2 in this volume, for an extensive description of stimulus overselectivity).

Unresponsivity and Neurological Development

A considerable body of experimental literature suggests that anatomical and physiological development can be drastically impaired by a variety of different types of unresponsivity to environmental stimulation (cf. Krech, Rosenzweig, & Bennett, 1966; Rosenzweig, 1976; Skuse, 1984; Wiesel & Hubel, 1965). For example, Greenough (1975) reviewed a number of studies showing that the formation of synaptic connections may not occur unless an adequate amount, variety, and complexity of environmental stimulation are provided. Also, Greenough, Volkmar, and Juraska (1973) showed that the extent and anatomical location of such impairments in dendritic branching are a function of the specific amount (moderate versus extreme deprivation) and type (e.g., visual, auditory, or motor) of deprivation (see also Neville, 1985).

Such impairments appear to occur in practically all advanced organisms and at practically all ages. It is important to note, however, that the devastating effects of deprivation may vary at different ages. For example, the neurological results of sensory deprivation are minimized if some responding to normal stimulation is provided first (e.g., Coleman & Riesen, 1968; Riesen, 1975; Valverde, 1967, 1971). It is also important to note that remediation of deprivation effects is greater if subsequent normal stimulation is provided at an early age (Baxter, 1969; Finger & Stein, 1982; Hubel, 1967; Hubel & Wiesel, 1970; Riesen, 1966, 1975; Walk & Gibson, 1961). The implications of such data are that early detection of sensory deprivation problems may be very important. Further, it implies that a prolonged period of sensory deprivation would be expected to change entire areas of the developmental sequence, and that such effects would be difficult to remediate without an early intervention (see also Wetherby, Koegel, & Mendel, 1981).

BEHAVIORAL IMPLICATIONS OF RESPONSIVITY

In addition to neurological studies such as those already described, there is a large body of literature discussing the importance of responding to environmental stimulation for direct improvements in behavior. Interactions with environmental stimuli have been shown to greatly improve not only neurological functioning but also specific and general learning. For example, natural consequences of specific environmental interactions can measurably improve learning about those specific stimuli and about the behaviors required to interact with such stimuli (cf. R. L. Koegel & Williams, 1980; Sailor & Taman, 1972; Skinner, 1979; Williams, Koegel, & Egel, 1981; etc.). For example, a child who is playing with a lunch box and accidentally opens the box to find a snack inside is likely to learn the specific responses necessary to manipulate the latch mechanism on the lunch box. Similarly, a child who accidentally touches a hot stove is likely to learn to be careful around stoves, and a child who repeatedly manipulates a toy puzzle is likely to learn how to assemble the puzzle. In addition, it also appears that children who engage in many such environmental interactions may develop generalized learning strategies, or actually "learn to learn" (Harlow, 1949). In contrast, a child who engages in very few and very perseverative interactions is likely to learn only a limited set of skills pertaining to the environment; and, further, is likely to have fewer generalized learning strategies for solving new or difficult problems. In extreme cases, the absence of natural consequences associated with limited responding may actually result in a "learned helplessness," with the individual actually becoming less and less responsive over time (see section following on motivation).

In addition to the impairments in neurological development and in learning caused by sensory deprivation, there also appear to be impairments in emotional development as well. For example, such individuals may score as highly anxious, hypersensitive, and irritable on psychological batteries (Toscher & Rupp, 1974). It also is interesting to note that normal human infants are generally active and irritable under conditions of relative stimulus deprivation (e.g., Bartoshuk, 1962; Birns, Blank, Bridger, & Escalona, 1965; Brackbill, Adams, Crowell, & Gray, 1966). Further, the presentation of certain types of stimulation (heartbeat, lullaby, metronome, etc.) will almost certainly quiet a restless child (Brackbill et al., 1966). Finally, it may be important to note that almost everyone who participates in sensory deprivation experiments reports the experience to be highly aversive and anxiety inducing (cf. Zubek, 1969).

Summary

Overall, the foregoing literature is representative of a large body of literature that suggests that sensory deprivation results in impairments in both neurological and behavioral development, and that the types of behaviors shown by autistic children (such as perseverative responding, restricted responding, responding primarily to single stimuli, etc.) would be expected to produce sensory deprivation effects. Further, such children's abnormal learning strategies, impaired motivation, abnormal emotional development, and so forth, are similar to the resulting behaviors described in the sensory deprivation literature. The remainder of this chapter, therefore, addresses techniques for remediating unresponsivity, based on the hypothesis that remediating autistic children's lack of responsivity would result in widespread improvements in their development. Two areas, increasing motivation and increasing self-monitoring skills, are each discussed in detail.

MOTIVATION: INCREASING RESPONDING

Description of the Problem

One of the problems in improving responsiveness relates to the fact that autistic children typically appear unmotivated to be responsive. Interestingly, a review of much of the research literature shows one striking parallel to such children's extreme lack of responding. This parallel is in the behavior of subjects who have participated in "learned helplessness" experiments (cf. R. L. Koegel & Egel, 1979; Seligman, 1972; Seligman, Klein, & Miller, 1976; Seligman, Maier, & Geer, 1968). Such subjects, when exposed to noncontingent reinforcement (which often parallels the type of natural consequences autistic children receive when they exhibit the abnormal responsiveness described here), become less and less motivated to remedy their plight. The problem appears to occur with both noncontingent positive and noncontingent aversive consequences. It appears that because consequences for responding are noncontingent, the individual learns that responding and reinforcement are not related, and future responding becomes lethargic. If this situation occurs on a continuous and frequent basis, the individual becomes severely unresponsive to environmental stimulation.

Learned Helplessness Hypothesis

As already noted, because of their abnormal responsivity, autistic and other severely handicapped children are often exposed to circumstances of noncontingent consequences in their natural environments. For example, a child who is putting on a jacket just as the school bus arrives, may end up with an adult buttoning the jacket so the child will not miss the bus. Paradoxically, the overall result of such an interaction may be that: 1) the child does not learn how to button the jacket and 2) the child experiences noncontingent "success" with respect to learning how to button the jacket. Also, because of their handicaps, such children are typically exposed to a very high density of failure for even attempting to learn new tasks. If such circumstances are very prevalent in the child's life, the authors postulate that a condition of "learned helplessness" would be likely to result, with a concomitant further decrease in overall responsivity to the environment.

Treatment of Motivation

Working from the hypothesis that autistic children's severe unresponsivity may be exacerbated because of a state of learned helplessness, a number of treatments have been developed in order to try to improve such children's motivation to respond to their environment. Some of the more prevalent areas of research are summarized in the next two subsections.

Prompt Successes   R. L. Koegel and Egel (1979), Churchill (1971), MacMillan (1971), and others have argued that treatment interventions designed to systematically increase exposure to response-reinforcer contingencies (between responding to a task and succeeding at that task) would be likely to improve autistic children's motivation to respond (as a pivotal response), and therefore would improve a wide range of their functioning.

For example, R. L. Koegel and Egel (1979) conducted an analysis (see Figure 1) of autistic children's responses to simple learning tasks, and found that: 1) the children usually failed at the tasks when left to themselves and 2) both the children's responding and enthusiasm decreased to extremely low levels if they were repeatedly exposed to the task that they were failing. However, designing treatment interventions to prompt the children to keep responding, and changing the initial task characteristics to raise the probability of an eventual correct response resulted in: 1) coincidental reinforcement for not only completing the task but also for responsivity per se and 2) subsequent increased levels of responsivity and enthusiasm for learning the tasks. Further, the results suggested that the children's overall learning strategies improved to the extent that rather large degrees of creative responding to new and difficult learning tasks began to occur.

The specific procedures used to accomplish these results relied on two strategies. First, the children were prompted to continue responding even if they were incorrect (for related studies, see also R. L. Koegel, O'Dell, & Dunlap, in press, and R. L. Koegel, O'Dell, & Koegel, 1987). Often a large variety of physical and verbal prompts (such as nudging or offering repeated verbal encouragement) was necessary in the early stages because the children frequently and aggressively attempted to cease responding to the task. Thus, a considerable amount of creativity typically was required on the therapist's part in order to maintain the children's responding during the early stages of this intervention. Second, during the initial treatment trials, the therapist arranged the learning task in such a way as to increase the probability of success. For example, a music box might be set to start playing music if the child placed

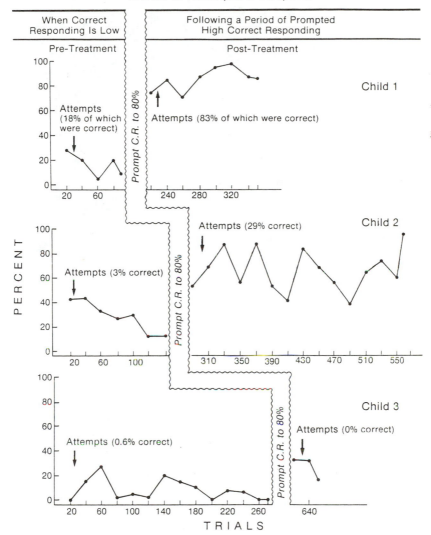

Figure 1.   The percentage of intervals with attempts at responding to the task during pre-treatment (when the children generally completed the task incorrectly) as compared with posttreatment, following a period of prompted correct responding (C.R.). (Reprinted with permission from Koegel, R.L., & Egel, A.L. [1979]. Motivating autistic children. *Journal of Abnormal Psychology, 88,* 418–426. Copyright 1979 by American Psychological Association, Inc.)

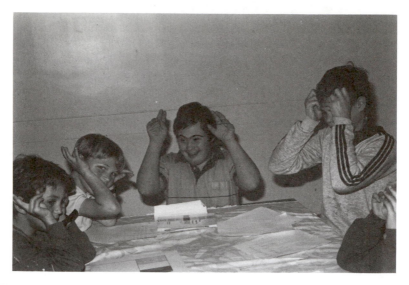

The child in the middle, who was previously lethargic, is now highly motivated to respond in instructional interactions in his classroom.

even a slight amount of pressure on the winding mechanism; or all of the holes except the relevant one in a geometric puzzle box might be taped shut, so that a child attempting to insert a geometric block into the box would be likely to succeed.

As the trials progressed throughout this treatment, two systematic changes were made in the therapist's behavior. First, therapist prompts for responsivity were systematically faded through a graduated guidance paradigm. As the number and variety of the children's responses increased, prompting responsivity eventually became unnecessary. Second, the type of task was systematically changed by the therapist so that task difficulty was ultimately increased to very difficult levels.

Intersperse Maintenance Tasks   As the preceding procedures were accomplished, the technique of interspersing numerous maintenance (previously acquired) tasks among the new learning trials was also utilized (see Dunlap, 1984; L. K. Koegel & Koegel, 1986; Neef, Iwata, & Page, 1980). This resulted in very high degrees of contingent reinforcement for responding during what ultimately became extremely difficult and sophisticated learning sessions for these children (see Figure 2). Koegel and Koegel now have continued this progression beyond that described in R. L. Koegel and Egel (1979), with the ultimate goal being to have children work on the extremely difficult task of remediating autism per se (cf. R. L. Koegel & Mentis, 1985). It is the authors' hypothesis that the extremely high number and variety of responses exhibited

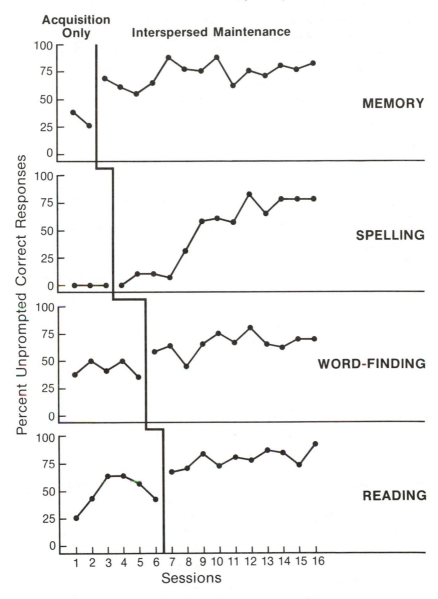

Figure 2.   Percentage of correct unprompted responses on acquisition tasks for the two conditions, acquisition tasks only versus acquisition tasks with interspersed maintenance tasks. (Reprinted with permission from Koegel, L.K., & Koegel, R.L. [1986]. The effects of interspersed maintenance tasks on academic performance in a severe childhood stroke victim. *Journal of Applied Behavior Analysis, 19,* 425–430. Copyright 1986 by The Society for the Experimental Analysis of Behavior.)

by the children in the latter stages of this treatment will result in improved neurological and behavioral functioning. The pilot data to date support this hypothesis and make the authors feel extremely encouraged about the long-term potential for this treatment approach. The benefits of this treatment approach (i.e., those of motivating durable and varied responsivity to the environment) are illustrated in the following description of a child in the authors' treatment program.

Case History: William

William, a boy who had many autistic characteristics, was extremely lethargic when he entered our clinic program at the age of 5. He typically lay down on his back on the floor and sucked his thumb, remaining practically impervious to all social and environmental stimuli. At that time, our research had not yet identified the importance of working on pivotal behaviors such as motivation, and William therefore participated in several years of more traditional treatment. By the time he was about 9 years old, motivation was still a serious problem, and his overall progress was extremely limited. However, by that time we had begun to realize the likely significance of targeting motivation as a pivotal behavior, and we therefore developed a "motivation" treatment program for William. The early stages of William's treatment, therefore, involved simple tasks such as teaching him to operate the music box and the puzzle box referred to earlier. As he learned to be responsive to those tasks, the difficulty level of subsequent tasks was gradually increased. As such, he was prompted to learn to dress himself by initially using clothing with large buttons and loose button holes, pants with elastic waistbands, shoes with partially tied laces, and so forth. On subsequent trials, the buttons were smaller, a belt was added to the pants, the shoes were untied further, and so on. The authors also worked on tasks in the area of recreation. For example, William was taught to hit a baseball with a bat by starting with a very soft and large ball, pitched to him slowly. Then a smaller ball was introduced, with the speed increased, and so forth. Throughout these sessions the child was constantly prompted to remain responsive and was reinforced for attempts to respond so that his motivation was always the focus of treatment as a pivotal target behavior. Eventually, by continuing to work on numerous such tasks, William's responsivity increased to the point where the authors felt he could be placed "on his own" in several community settings. Initially, he was taken to a pizza parlor with some money and was instructed to purchase a pizza and a large soft drink. He was then left "on his own" to accomplish this task (although the therapist was covertly close enough to assist should an emergency arise). William's first obstacle was to discover that he needed to stand in line to order the pizza. Initially, he attempted to go to the front of the line. However, as he received a certain amount of guidance from other customers, he eventually learned the appropriate way to wait in line for his turn. Then, because his articulation was very poor, it took him a fairly extended amount of time to explain his order to the clerk. He was repeatedly questioned by the clerk, and had to respond numerous times until she eventually figured out what he wanted. Ultimately, however, he was able to successfully place his order, pay for it, and take the food to a table and eat. Although this may seem like a relatively simple endeavor for most, it involved numerous complex behaviors that were not conducive to training in a clinical setting, such as standing in line, deciding on the size of the pizza and on what kind of soft drink, and so on. Thus, numerous unexpected incidental behaviors were acquired as a result of targeting the pivotal behavior of motivation. Anecdotally, it is interesting to note that William also placed an additional order for another soft drink and gave it to a girl who was seated near him. In addition, he obtained napkins and straws, and cleaned the table after he was finished eating. He also picked up some wayward papers from the ground and threw them into the trash container as he walked back to the clinic. These were all spontaneous child behaviors that were not trained in the clinic.

From a treatment perspective, it is important to note that an extremely large and varied number of responses occurred during the foregoing task. The child made numerous, varied, and creative verbal and nonverbal responses over an extended period of time. Further, many natural reinforcers occurred as a result of his appropriate responding, thus increasing his exposure to favorable response-reinforcer contingencies. The literature and the research in the authors' laboratory suggest that this is resulting in direct improvements in: 1) neurological development (i.e., William's electroencephalograms have significantly normalized since he began treatment); 2) direct task learning (shoe tying, buttoning clothes, restaurant skills, etc., have all improved); 3) general learning strategies (he appears to learn novel tasks more quickly); 4) social and emotional development (he appears happier and more interested in people); and 5) motivation to attempt new learning tasks (i.e., William now attempts to respond in even very difficult, new learning situations). Overall, the extremely widespread extent of such improvements is expected to continue producing dramatic and continuous alterations in the child's development.

UNRESPONSIVITY ACROSS MULTIPLE ENVIRONMENTS

Description of the Problem

Another problem in the treatment of children with autism or other disabilities is that generalization of treatment gains to nontreatment environments frequently does not occur (Baer, Wolf, & Risley, 1968; Kazdin & Bootzin, 1972; R. L.

Koegel & Rincover, 1977). Often, treatment programs focus primarily on behavioral change within the treatment setting. Therefore, while responsivity may be improved within the treatment setting, there is still not likely to be enough overall responding throughout the day to produce the requisite types of neurological and behavioral changes suggested earlier. Thus, the lack of generalization can cause devastating effects for both the child and significant others in the child's environment (R. L. Koegel & Koegel, 1987). Many researchers and practitioners now realize the importance of focusing on behaviors that will be likely to generalize, as has been discussed, and of incorporating generalization activities as an integral part of the treatment program (Costello, 1983). Without such activities, the entire treatment program may be of little value to the child. A brief review of several other methods that have been useful in promoting generalization appears next, followed by a discussion of the use of self-monitoring as a pivotal behavior. Self-monitoring procedures can be used either as a tool to promote generalization of individual target behaviors trained in the clinical setting or to measure and reward "motivation" (i.e., increased responsivity) in environments that may not support its occurrence.

Treatment of Generalization

Numerous treatment techniques have been discussed in the literature, and many have been very useful in either promoting generalized responsivity directly or providing a sound basis for further research. Some of these techniques can be conducted entirely within the clinical setting. For example, including functional and salient stimuli (Stokes & Baer, 1977), such as pictures and objects, that occur in the child's natural environment is likely to promote generalized responsivity in new settings (Costello, 1977). This is because the relevant stimuli may serve as a discriminative stimulus and may evoke the target behavior in the natural environment. Generalization can also be accomplished by bringing in relevant stimuli from the child's environment such as class work, toys, parents, or even peers (cf. Johnston & Johnston, 1972). Also, using a large number of stimuli may serve to widen the conditions under which the response will occur (Stokes & Baer, 1977) and may help to increase the possibility that the response will occur even if the stimulus item does not exactly replicate the natural environment (Spradlin & Siegel, 1982). Finally, overpractice and practicing the newly learned behavior with increased speed (Bankson & Byrne, 1972; Fitts, 1965) are likely to promote generalization outside of the treatment setting.

Other techniques designed to promote generalized responsivity can be programmed outside of the clinical setting. For example, sequential modification, such as training in multiple environments or training another individual to provide treatment in a setting beyond the clinic, has been shown to be effective (Griffiths & Craighead, 1972; Murdock, Garcia, & Hardman, 1977). Training "significant others" to implement the treatment, such as a parent (Costello & Bosler, 1976; Raver, Cooke, & Apolloni, 1978; Wing & Heimgartner, 1973), peers (Bailey, Timbers, Phillips, & Wolf, 1971), or other paraprofessionals (Costello & Schoen, 1978; Galloway & Blue, 1975), has also been shown to be very effective in promoting use of the newly learned behavior in the child's natural environment (see Fowler, Chapter 7, in this volume).

SELF-MANAGEMENT PROCEDURES

Another method of promoting generalized responsivity across multiple settings that is receiving much attention is the use of self-management procedures. Self-management procedures appear to incorporate many of the individual techniques described earlier (also see discussion following), which may contribute to its effectiveness. The use of self-management strategies can be time efficient (Fowler, 1984) and also can be trained within the clinical setting, which is usually a convenient and controlled setting without competing distractions. In addition, self-management procedures are easy to implement and require few special materials (R. L. Koegel, Koegel, & Ingham, 1986). Finally, and probably most importantly, the procedures allow the child to functionally serve as his or her own therapist. This in turn, reduces the need for constant teacher vigilance and can recruit the use of newly acquired behaviors during unsupervised activities (cf. Fowler, 1984).

Self-Management as a Pivotal Target Behavior

It is important to note that many researchers and theorists consider the absence of self-monitoring skills to be a pivotal deficit in normal development. The purpose of this portion of the chapter, therefore, is to discuss teaching the use of self-management strategies as a pivotal target behavior. That is, by teaching the children the "skill" of self-management as a pivotal behavior, an indefinite number of behaviors can be targeted in virtually any environment the child enters. Such widespread changes in responsivity have the potential to be large enough to produce changes in both neurological functioning and general learning strategies.

Self-management procedures can also be very effective if used in combination with the motivational treatment described earlier. That is, the generalized responsivity that also results from focusing on motivation can be systematically programmed and rewarded in the child's natural environment through the use of self-management techniques.

General Steps

Self-management procedures can be conducted in a variety of ways, emphasizing some or all of the components (e.g., self-monitoring, self-reinforcement) of the general paradigm. The procedures utilized in the authors' work have focused primarily on the child's self-monitoring of appropriate behavior, with reinforcers provided to a large extent by external sources (up to the point where natural reinforcers might be expected to begin taking effect). As such, the remainder of this chapter focuses on describing the child's use of self-monitoring procedures as a pivotal behavior that influences responding across a wide variety of natural environments.

Following the successful implementation of several speech programs using self-monitoring techniques (see L. K. Koegel & Koegel, 1983, 1986; R. L. Koegel et al., 1986), the authors were able to extrapolate some general steps that would later serve as the basis for the development of a variety of self-monitoring programs. These general steps are divided into four categories: 1) preparation for the training of self-monitoring, 2) training self-monitoring, 3) evaluating and rewarding self-monitoring behavior that occurs in the natural environment, and 4) fading the formal self-monitoring activities.

During the preparation stage, the treatment and generalization settings are specifically defined. Also, both inappropriate behaviors and appropriate target responses are defined. Functional rewards, chosen by the child, are delineated and an appropriate period of time or unit of behavior that will be small enough to result in success on the child's part is determined.

Following the preparatory steps, the clinician begins training self-monitoring. In order to do this, the child is taught to discriminate between the correct versus the incorrect behavior. With many populations this can be accomplished through modeling and requiring the child to demonstrate the behaviors, to be sure that the child has learned the discrimination. If the child is more severely handicapped, it may be possible to begin by simply prompting the child to engage in the appropriate behavior.

Next, the child is taught to self-observe, self-evaluate, and then record the fact that a unit of behavior has taken place. A number of self-evaluation programs have been developed that range from recording a plus (+) or a check mark following each occurrence of the correct target behavior (R. L. Koegel et al., 1986) to evaluating one's own behavior during a specific time period, then rating that period of behavior on a predetermined scale (e.g., Rhode, Morgan, & Young, 1983). Following successful completion to an individual criterion that assures the clinician that the child is able to perform the activities, the child is prompted to perform the self-monitoring activities under appropriate natural stimulus conditions. It should be noted that if the self-monitoring is not programmed to occur under relevant stimulus conditions within the child's natural environment, it is not likely that the appropriate behavior will generalize within any practical period of time (R. L. Koegel, Koegel, Van Voy, & Ingham, in press).

After the child has been instructed to perform the monitoring in a specific environment, the clinician validates that the self-monitoring behaviors have indeed occurred in the desired environment(s). This can be accomplished by checking with "significant others" in the child's environment, then either prompting the behavior if it is not occurring, implementing a contingency if the child is turning in points without actually performing the appropriate behavior, or administering the rewards if appropriate behavior and monitoring are occurring.

Finally, the last phase of the program, fading the formal self-monitoring activities, is implemented. This can be accomplished in several ways, including gradually increasing the number of points required for a reward, lengthening the time period of appropriate behavior required for a reward, increasing the behavioral unit needed to earn an award, or in some cases by simply telling the child that because he or she is doing so well the self-monitoring is no longer necessary. The following two case histories illustrate some of the authors' experiences in developing self-monitoring programs.

Case History: John

John, a 5-year-old boy, was referred to the authors by his preschool teachers for the treatment of autisticlike behaviors. A behavioral assessment conducted by the authors indicated that he demonstrated numerous inappropriate behaviors

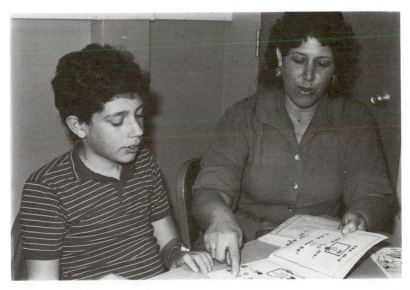

The child is engaged in a conversational activity with his mother. Note the wrist counter for monitoring appropriate conversational responses.

including tantrums, aggression, inappropriate play, inappropriate social skills, lack of appropriate emotions (e.g., excessive crying) and inappropriate use of language skills. He also had obsessions with specific toys and small objects. Although his inappropriate behaviors made him extremely difficult to test, his IQ was estimated at 50 on nonverbal IQ tests.

John's special education treatment provider decided that self-monitoring would be an excellent pivotal behavior for him to acquire for application to his numerous inappropriate behaviors across a wide variety of stimulus situations. That is, the very large numbers of behaviors and settings with impaired responsivity appeared to be placing this child in a functionally sensory impoverished environment. Therefore, one would expect it to be extremely difficult to produce any clinically significant developmental changes in this child's functioning unless a procedure could be devised to target a large number of behaviors across a large number of stimulus conditions. Self-monitoring seemed an ideal avenue for this goal.

After initial work on establishing appropriate sitting and attending skills within the clinic, the authors began to focus on generalized appropriate responding through the use of self-monitoring activities. Once John was able to successfully complete a few consecutive trials, training began on self-monitoring. Because, as mentioned earlier, John had no previous formal education, behaviors that would be useful for the self-monitoring program—such as holding and using a pencil, the use of a token system, and basic concepts such as full versus empty—were incorporated into the sessions.

The self-monitoring training began with the following preparation. First, John's existing inappropriate behaviors and the desired appropriate behaviors were defined. The list of inappropriate behaviors was lengthy, ranging from major interfering behaviors such as tantrums, to less obtrusive behaviors such as staring into space. His appropriate behaviors included sitting quietly within the learning setting, facing forward at the table with his eyes on the clinician or task materials, and his hands held appropriately without interfering self-stimulatory behavior. Targeting such behaviors seemed likely to permit a large increase in responding to the types of learning stimuli that would result in a sensory enriched environment.

John chose several commercially purchased "scratch and sniff" stickers to earn as rewards. These were able to be exchanged for tokens (i.e., the happy faces discussed in the next paragraph), which were administered along with social praise and could serve as intermediary reinforcers. Finally, it was necessary to determine an appropriate period of time for John to begin self-monitoring. Because he had no prior experience with any type of self-monitoring program or systematic behavioral management, and because he was functioning at a severely handicapped level, the authors decided to begin with a very short (10-

second) period of time in order to maximize the likelihood of success on John's part, in the hope that his motivation to learn would also improve.

Next, the authors trained John to evaluate his own behavior. First the authors drew one box on a small (3 in. × 5 in.) piece of paper. Then the authors modeled and verbally labeled both appropriate and inappropriate behavior, and drew a happy or sad face, respectively, immediately following the demonstration. The clinician then modeled the receipt of a sticker (reward) following the occurrence of appropriate behavior. Next, the authors prompted John to monitor his own behavior. A very short time period for monitoring (10 seconds) was chosen, in order to increase the likelihood of success, and, as suspected, John was able to behave appropriately for that period of time. Next, the authors guided John through the process of recording a happy face on the small sheet of paper and then comparing it to the clinician's evaluation in order to validate his accuracy. He then received his reward following agreement between both clinician and child.

After several successful trials, the authors began to decrease the frequency of the rewards being given by the clinician. This was accomplished in a twofold manner: 1) the number of tokens (happy faces) required to receive a reward was increased and 2) the time period between recordings was lengthened. This was accomplished very gradually and systematically. If the time period was lengthened too rapidly and resulted in several consecutive periods of inappropriate behavior, the time period was shortened again in order to ensure success. Eventually, John was able to behave appropriately for 15-minute intervals and to earn six happy faces per sticker (thus behaving appropriately for 1½ hours for each sticker).

The next step was to prompt and reinforce the occurrence of self-monitoring under the relevant natural stimulus conditions in John's classroom environment. Specifically, since the goal for this child was appropriate behavior under a wide variety of classroom stimulus conditions, the monitoring was prompted and reinforced in the classroom (i.e., outside of the clinical setting) by his special education treatment provider, who also continued to provide rewards for the points John turned in during his regular clinic sessions. Thus, John was prompted to monitor appropriate responding in areas such as the library section of the room, where he began to look at the books instead of throwing them or ignoring them. He was also prompted to monitor his behavior in the animal section of the room, where he began to observe and label the various animals, as well as in the toy area, the cloakroom area, the music section, and so forth. In each case, instead of throwing a tantrum or staring into space, John began to interact with the relevant stimulus materials in an appropriate way, resulting in further learning and therefore more opportunities for responsivity. It is interesting to note here that the implementation of the self-monitoring activities directly improved John's overall responsivity in his natural environment without specific training. For example, he also began to help clean up toys and equipment in his classroom environment. This was a typical behavior performed by his nonhandicapped peers, but required actual observation and modeling for John to learn.

As of this writing, the program just described is working extremely well under conditions that are maintained by occasional external reinforcers provided by the clinician. The authors ultimate goal, however, will be to fade reliance on both the external reinforcers and the self-monitoring activities, and to attempt to rely more on natural social reinforcers from John's peers and teachers.

Case History: Danny

Danny, a 12-year-old autistic boy, who was also legally deaf and visually impaired, was referred to us because of severe hygiene problems. His parents went to work before he woke up in the morning, and were unable to supervise his hygiene before he left for school on the bus. Therefore, self-management procedures seemed an ideal way to promote Danny's responsivity with respect to hygiene skills in this and other unsupervised settings. To begin his self-monitoring program, the authors performed an observation in Danny's natural environment and behaviorally defined his inappropriate behaviors (Johnson & Koegel, 1982). This resulted in numerous behaviors identified as in need of remediation, including "dirty face," "dirty glasses," "dirty hair," and so on. In addition, he exhibited the "sameness" tendency often seen in people with autism (Ritvo & Freeman, 1978) and repeatedly wore the same pants, shirt and socks, resulting in extremely dirty and foul-smelling clothes.

Because numerous previous attempts to work on hygiene as an overall target behavior were unsuccessful, the authors worked on one behavior at a time as determined by Danny's behavioral assessment (cf. Cone & Hawkins, 1977). Cleaning his face was the first behavior chosen because it was easily observable and could be remediated at home as well as school, if necessary. To complete the preparatory stage, the desired outcome for this subskill was defined as follows: the child's face contains no observable dirt, other markings or mucous in his eyes. Finally, a functional positive reinforcer (going to the park with the clinician) was chosen by the child.

Training Danny to self-monitor began in a small clinical room that contained a sink and a mirror. Danny was prompted to look in the mirror to evaluate the condition of his face. If it was dirty, he was prompted to wash it, and then to evaluate it again. Immediately after evaluating his face, he was instructed to mark a check on a piece of paper if his face was clean. This was repeated on several different days. Then the therapist took him to his home and guided him through the process at his own sink. Next, Danny was instructed to complete the process daily, prior to leaving for school, and was told that after seven successful days he could earn his reward.

In order to validate his monitoring, either Danny's clinician or teacher met the bus periodically to evaluate the accuracy of his monitoring. If his face was clean and he had marked a check in his book, he was verbally reinforced and received a point toward his tangible reward. If his face was dirty and he had not marked a point, he was verbally reinforced for accurate monitoring, and was then taken to the clinical room to wash his face, but he did not receive a point. If he performed inaccurate monitoring, he received no points at all, and he was verbally reprimanded.

Finally, it was necessary to fade the monitoring system to more closely approximate the conditions required by the natural environment. This was accomplished in two ways: first, after several additional successful days were completed, one more behavior was targeted so that Danny received one point daily for the two target behaviors successfully completed and accurately monitored. This was repeated until all of the behaviors were eventually included. In addition, the number of points required to receive the tangible reward was gradually increased. Once this very thin schedule of reinforcement was achieved, the natural reinforcement of approval from peers and teachers appeared to maintain appropriate responding without the need for further self-monitoring activities. It is interesting to note that Danny ultimately demonstrated a more generalized responsivity by adding several new behaviors to his repertoire, such as wearing a tie to school, thus demonstrating the more widespread type of responsivity that the authors had been hoping for. He also began to self-monitor and to exhibit appropriate hygiene behavior when he stayed at his grandmother's home, even though that setting had not been specifically targeted. Overall, his entire program was completed in about 3 months, a relatively short period of time compared to the several years during which his poor hygiene skills had presented a problem. Thus, one pivotal behavior, self-monitoring, was able to rapidly and successfully mediate numerous other behaviors in numerous unsupervised settings, creating a high level of favorable environmental interactions.

Overview of Self-Monitoring

Both of these case examples, and the literature in general, document the effectiveness of self-monitoring procedures for decreasing inappropriate behaviors, and therefore for indirectly increasing the opportunity for appropriate environmental responding (Gardner, Clees, & Cole, 1983; Gardner, Cole, Berry, & Norwinski, 1983; Reese, Sherman, & Sheldon, 1984), as well as for increasing or improving appropriate responding directly (Anderson-Inman, Paine, &

Deutchman, 1984; Baer, Fowler, & Carden-Smith, 1984; R. L. Koegel et al., 1986; McNally, Dompile, & Sherman, 1984; Shapiro, Browder, & D'Huyvetters, 1984).

The widespread success of self-monitoring programs on these numerous behaviors may be attributed to several different variables. First, as mentioned at the beginning of this chapter, many factors that are included in our self-monitoring programs have previously been shown to be successful in promoting generalization. For example, issues related to reinforcement, such as the administration of delayed rewards (Dunlap, Koegel, Johnson, & O'Neill, 1987) and of unpredictable rewards (Dunlap & Johnson, 1985; R. L. Koegel & Rincover, 1977), have been shown to promote steady, durable levels of responding, and are included in many self-monitoring programs. Second, the visibility of the self-monitoring, and/or the occurrence or improvement of the target behavior, may encourage other individuals in the natural environment to provide reinforcers (Baer et al., 1984), initiating a favorable cycle of steadily improving environmental interactions. A third variable may relate to the stimulus control of the recording device. That is, because the device has been paired with reinforcement, it is likely to acquire stimulus control for the occurrence or improvement of the desired target behaviors (Liberty, 1983; Nelson & Hayes, 1981). Other factors discussed by Stokes and Baer (1977) that may contribute to generalization, and that are also included in many self-monitoring programs, are loose training, including multiple exemplars, and training in multiple environments.

Finally, client variables, such as IQ (Bornstein, 1985), cognitive stage (Barkley, Copeland, & Savage, 1980; Schleser, Cohen, Meyers, & Rodrick, 1984); and motivation (Engel, Brandriet, Erickson, Gronhovd, & Gunderson, 1966; Komaki & Dore-Boyce, 1978; Powers, 1971) have been discussed as influencing the success of the procedures. Thus, improvements in each of these areas would be expected to further increase the effectiveness of the programs, producing an escalating cycle of improvements. All of these areas need to be researched further to gain more knowledge into their effectiveness. However, at this point, enough information already appears to be known to produce widespread appropriate responding across numerous natural environments.

SUMMARY

This chapter has discussed two types of pivotal behaviors, motivation to respond to environmental stimuli (i.e., increasing responsivity) and self-monitoring of responsivity, both of which may be utilized to change numerous responses across numerous settings, resulting in more widespread developmental improvements in severely handicapped individuals. These methods have been developed in hopes that they will replace the need for lengthy clinical programs devoted to the individual remediation of incredibly large numbers of separate target behaviors. The resultant large change in the affected children's overall responsivity to their environment is postulated to produce major developmental changes in both neurological functioning and general learning. This may be accomplished through the use of pivotal target behaviors, which encourage the children to "be their own therapists" and to thereby take responsibility for the multitude of behaviors in need of being affected. Such an approach now seems necessary if we are to expect widespread and durable behavior changes in very severely handicapped individuals.

REFERENCES

Anderson-Inman, L., Paine, S.C., & Deutchman, L. (1984). Neatness counts: Effects of direct instruction and self-monitoring on the transfer of neat-paper skills to non-training settings. *Analysis and Intervention in Developmental Disabilities, 4*(2), 137–156.

Anthony, J. (1958). An experimental approach to the psychopathology of childhood autism. *British Journal of Medical Psychology, 31,* 211–225.

Baer, D.M., Wolf, M.M., & Risley, T.R. (1968). Some current dimensions of applied behavior analysis. *Journal of Applied Behavior Analysis, 1,* 91–97.

Baer, M., Fowler, S.A., & Carden-Smith, L. (1984). Using reinforcement and independent-grading to promote and maintain task accuracy in a mainstreamed class. *Analysis and Intervention in Developmental Disabilities, 4*(2), 157–170.

Bailey, J.S., Timbers, G.D., Phillips, E.L., & Wolf, M.M. (1971). Modification of articulation errors by pre-delinquents by their peers. *Journal of Applied Behavior Analysis, 4,* 265–281.

Bankson, N.W., & Byrne, M.C. (1972). The effect of a timed correct sound production task on carryover. *Journal of Speech and Hearing Research, 15,* 160–168.

Barkley, R.A., Copeland, A.P., & Savage, C. (1980). A self-control classroom for hyperactive children. *Journal of Autism and Developmental Disorders, 10,* 75–89.

Bartoshuk, A.K. (1962). Response decrement with repeated elicitation of human neonatal cardiac acceleration to sound. *Journal of Comparative and Physiological Psychology, 55,* 9–13.

Baxter, B.L. (1969). Effect of visual deprivation during postnatal maturation on the electroencephalogram of a cat. *Experimental Neurology, 14,* 224–237.

Birns, B., Blank, M., Bridger, W.H., & Escalona, S.K. (1965). Behavioral inhibition of neonates produced by auditory stimuli. *Child Development, 36,* 639–645.

Bornstein, P.H. (1985). Self-instructional training: A commentary and state of the art. *Journal of Applied Behavior Analysis, 18,* 69–72.

Brackbill, Y., Adams, G., Crowell, D.H., & Gray, M.L. (1966). Arousal level in neonates and preschool children under continuous auditory stimulation. *Journal of Experimental Child Psychology, 4,* 178–188.

Churchill, D.W. (1971). Effects of success and failure in psychotic children. *Archives of General Psychology, 25,* 208–214.

Coleman, P.D., & Riesen, A.H. (1968). Environmental effects on cortical dendritic fields: I. Rearing in the dark. *Journal of Anatomy, 102*, 363–374.

Cone, J.D., & Hawkins, R.D. (1977). *Behavioral assessment*. New York: Brunner/ Mazel.

Costello, J.M. (1977). Programmed instruction. *Journal of Speech and Hearing Disorders, 42*, 3–28.

Costello, J.M. (1983). Generalization across settings: Language intervention with children. In J. Miller, D.E. Yoder, & R. Schiefelbusch (Eds.), Contemporary issues in language intervention. *American Speech and Hearing Association Reports, 12*, 275–297.

Costello, J., & Bosler, S. (1976). Generalization and articulation instruction. *Journal of Speech and Hearing Disorders, 41*, 359–373.

Costello, J., & Schoen, J. (1978). The effectiveness of paraprofessionals and a speech clinician as agents of articulation intervention using programmed instruction. *Language, Speech, and Hearing Services in Schools, 9*, 118–128.

Dunlap, G. (1984). The influence of task variation and maintenance tasks on the learning and affect of autistic children. *Journal of Experimental Child Psychology, 37*, 41–64.

Dunlap, G., & Johnson, J. (1985). Increasing the independent responding of autistic children with unpredictable supervision. *Journal of Applied Behavior Analysis, 18*, 227–236.

Dunlap, G., Koegel, R.L., Johnson, J., & O'Neill, R.E. (1987). Maintaining performance of autistic clients in community settings with delayed contingencies. *Journal of Applied Behavior Analysis, 20*, 185–191.

Engel, D.C., Brandriet, S., Erickson, K., Gronhovd, K.D., & Gunderson, G. (1966). Carryover. *Journal of Speech and Hearing Disorders, 31*, 227–233.

Finger, S., & Stein, D.G. (1982). *Brain damage and recovery: Research and clinical perspectives*. New York: Academic Press.

Fiske, D.W., & Maddi, S.R. (1961). *Functions of varied experience*. Homewood, IL: Dorsey.

Fitts, P. (1965). Factors in complex skill training. In R. Glaser (Ed.), *Training research and education* (pp. 177–197). New York: John Wiley & Sons.

Fowler, S. (1984). Introductory comments: The pragmatics of self-management for the developmentally disabled. *Analysis and Intervention in Developmental Disabilities, 4*, 85–89.

Galloway, H.F., & Blue, J.M. (1975). Paraprofessional personnel in articulation therapy. *Language, Speech, and Hearing Services in Schools, 6*, 125–130.

Gardner, W.I., Clees, T.J., & Cole, C.L. (1983). Self-management of disruptive verbal ruminations by a mentally retarded adult. *Applied Research in Mental Retardation, 4*, 41–58.

Gardner, W.I., Cole, C.L., Berry, D.L., & Norwinski, J.M. (1983). Reduction of disruptive behaviors in mentally retarded adults: A self-management approach. *Behavior Modification, 7*, 76–96.

Greenough, W.T. (1975). Experimental modification of the developing brain. *American Scientist, 63*, 59–65.

Greenough, W.T. (1984). Structural correlates of information storage in the mammalian brain: A review and hypothesis. *Trends in Neurosciences, 7*, 229–233.

Greenough, W.T., Volkmar, F.R., & Juraska, J.M. (1973). Effects of rearing complexity on dendritic branching in frontolateral and temporal cortex of the rat. *Experimental*

Neurology, 41, 371–378.

Greer, E.R., Diamond, M.D., & Tang, J.M.W. (1982). Environmental enrichment in Brattleboro rats: Brain morphology. *Annals of the New York Academy of Sciences, 394,* 749–752.

Griffiths, H., & Craighead, W.E. (1972). Generalization in operant speech therapy. *Journal of Speech and Hearing Disorders, 37,* 485–494.

Harlow, H.F. (1949). The formation of learning sets. *Psychology Review, 56,* 51–65.

Hubel, D.H. (1967). Effects of distortion of sensory input on the visual system of kittens. *Physiologist, 10,* 17–45.

Hubel, D.H., & Wiesel, T.N. (1970). The period of susceptibility to the physiological effects of unilateral eye closure in kittens. *Journal of Physiology, 206,* 419–436.

Johnson, J., & Koegel, R.L. (1982). Behavioral assessment and curriculum development. In R.L. Koegel, A. Rincover, & A.L. Egel (Eds.), *Educating and understanding autistic children* (pp. 1–32). San Diego: College-Hill Press.

Johnston, J.M., & Johnston, G.T. (1972). Modification of consonant speech-sound articulation in young children. *Journal of Applied Behavioral Analysis, 5,* 233–246.

Kanner, L. (1943). Autistic disturbances of affective contact. *Nervous Child, 3,* 217–250.

Kazdin, A., & Bootzin, R.R. (1972). The token economy: An evaluative review. *Journal of Applied Behavior Analysis, 5,* 343–372.

Koegel, L.K., & Koegel, R.L. (1983). *How to program generalization of articulation gains through self-monitoring procedures. Field manual.* Santa Barbara: University of California, Santa Barbara.

Koegel, L.K, & Koegel, R.L. (1986). The effects of interspersed maintenance tasks on academic performance in a severe childhood stroke victim. *Journal of Applied Behavior Analysis, 19,* 425–430.

Koegel, R.L., & Egel, A.L. (1979). Motivating autistic children. *Journal of Abnormal Psychology, 88,* 4118–4126.

Koegel, R.L., & Felsenfeld, S. (1977). Sensory deprivation. In S. Gerber (Ed.), *Audiometry in infancy* (pp. 247–262). New York: Grune & Stratton.

Koegel, R.L., & Koegel, L.K. (1987). Generalization issues in the treatment of autism. *Seminars in Speech and Language.* New York: Thieme-Stratton.

Koegel, R.L., Koegel, L.K., & Ingham, J.C. (1986). Programming rapid generalization of correct articulation through self-monitoring procedures. *Journal of Speech and Hearing Disorders, 51,* 24–32.

Koegel, R.L., Koegel, L.K., Van Voy, K.G., & Ingham, J.C. (in press). In-clinic versus out-of-clinic self-monitoring of articulation to promote generalization. *Journal of Speech and Hearing Disorders.*

Koegel, R.L., & Mentis, M. (1985). Motivation in childhood autism: Can they or won't they? *Journal of Child Psychology and Psychiatry, 26,* 185–191.

Koegel, R.L., O'Dell, M.C., & Dunlap, G. (in press). Motivating speech use in nonverbal autistic children by reinforcing attempts. *Journal of Autism and Developmental Disorders.*

Koegel, R.L., O'Dell, M.C., & Koegel, L.K. (1987). A natural language teaching paradigm for nonverbal autistic children. *Journal of Autism and Developmental Disorders, 17,* 187–200.

Koegel, R.L., & Rincover, A. (1977). Some research on the difference between generalization and maintenance in extra-therapy settings. *Journal of Applied Behavior Analysis, 10,* 1–16.

Koegel, R.L., & Williams, J. (1980). Direct vs. indirect response-reinforcer relationships in teaching autistic children. *Journal of Abnormal Child Psychology, 4,* 537–547.

Komaki, J., & Dore-Boyce, K. (1978). Self-recording: Its effectiveness on individuals' high and low motivation. *Behavior Therapy, 9,* 65–72.

Krech, D., Rosenzweig, M.R., & Bennett, E. (1966). Environmental impoverishment, social isolation, and changes in brain chemistry and anatomy. *Physiology and Behavior, 1,* 99–104.

Liberty, K.A. (1983). Self-monitoring and skill generalization: A review of current research. In N.G. Haring, K. Liberty, F. Billingsley, O. While, V. Lynch, J. Kayser, & F. McCarthy (Eds.), *Investigating the problems of skill generalization* (pp. 37–53). Seattle: University of Washington Research Organization.

Lovaas, O.I., Koegel, R.L., & Schreibman, L. (1979). Stimulus overselectivity and autism: A review of research. *Psychological Bulletin, 86,* 1236–1254.

MacMillan, D.L. (1971). The problem of motivation in the education of the mentally retarded. *Exceptional Children, 37,* 579–586.

McNally, R.J., Dompile, J.J., & Sherman, G. (1984). Increasing the productivity of mentally retarded workers through self-management. *Analysis and Intervention in Developmental Disabilities, 4*(2), 129–136.

Murdock, J.Y., Garcia, E.E., & Hardman, M.L. (1977). Generalizing articulation training with trainable mentally retarded subjects. *Journal of Applied Behavior Analysis, 10,* 717–733.

Neef, N.A., Iwata, B.A., & Page, T.J. (1980). The effects of interspersal training versus high density reinforcement on spelling acquisition and retention. *Journal of Applied Behavior Analysis, 13,* 153–158.

Nelson, R.O., & Hayes, S.C. (1981). Theoretical explanations for reactivity in self-monitoring. *Behavior Modification, 5,* 3–14.

Neville, H.J. (1985). Effects of early sensory and language experience on the development of the human brain. In J. Mehler & R. Foxx (Eds.), *Neonate cognition: Beyond the blooming buzzing confusion* (pp. 349–364). Hillsdale, NJ: Lawrence Erlbaum Associates.

O'Neill, R. (1987). *Environmental interactions of normal children and children with autism.* Unpublished dissertation, University of California, Santa Barbara.

Ornitz, E.M (1974). The modulation of sensory input and motor output in autistic children. *Journal of Autism and Childhood Schizophrenia, 4,* 197–215.

Powers, M.H. (1971). Clinical and educational procedures in functional disorders of articulation. In L.H. Travis (Ed.), *Handbook of speech pathology and audiology* (pp. 877–910). New York: Appleton-Century-Crofts.

Raver, S.A., Cooke, T.P., & Apolloni, T. (1978). Generalization effects from intratherapy articulation: A case study. *Journal of Applied Behavior Analysis, 11,* 436.

Reese, M.R., Sherman, J.A., & Sheldon, J. (1984). Reducing agitated-disruptive behavior of mentally retarded residents of community group homes: The role of self-recording and peer prompted self-recording. *Analysis and Intervention in Developmental Disabilities, 4*(2), 91–108.

Rhode, G., Morgan, D.P., & Young, K.R. (1983). Generalization and maintenance of treatment gains of behaviorally handicapped students from resource rooms to regular classrooms using self-evaluation procedures. *Journal of Applied Behavior Analysis, 16,* 171–188.

Riesen, A.H. (1966). Sensory deprivation. In E. Stellar & J.M. Sprague (Eds.), *Prog-

ress in physiological psychology (pp. 117–142). New York: Academic Press.

Riesen, A.H. (1975). (Ed.), *The developmental neuropsychology of sensory deprivation*. New York: Academic Press.

Riesen, A.H., & Zilbert, D.E. (1975). Behavioral consequences of variations in early sensory environments. In A.H. Riesen (Ed.), *The developmental neuropsychology of sensory deprivation* (pp. 211–246). New York: Academic Press.

Ritvo, E.R., & Freeman, B.J. (1978). National Society for Autistic Children definition of the syndrome of autism. *Journal of Autism and Childhood Schizophrenia, 8,* 162–167.

Rosenzweig, M.R. (1976). Effects of environment on brain and behavior in animals. In E. Schopler & R.J. Reichler (Eds.), *Psychopathology and child development* (pp. 33–50). New York: Plenum.

Sailor, W., & Taman, T. (1972). Stimulus factors in the training of prepositional usage in three autistic children. *Journal of Applied Behavior Analysis, 5,* 183–192.

Schleser, R., Cohen, R., Meyers, A.W., & Rodick, J.D. (1984). The effects of cognition level and training on the generalization of self-instruction. *Cognitive Therapy and Research, 6,* 187–200.

Schopler, E. (1965). Early infantile autism and the receptor process. *Archives of General Psychiatry, 13,* 327–335.

Seligman, M.E.P. (1972). Learned helplessness. *Annual Review of Medicine, 23,* 407–412.

Seligman, M.E.P., Klein, D.D., & Miller, W.R. (1976). Depression. In H. Leitenberg (Ed.), *Handbook of behavior modification* (pp. 168–210). New York: Appleton-Century-Crofts.

Seligman, M.E.P., Maier, S.F., & Geer, J. (1968). The alleviation of learned helplessness in the dog. *Journal of Abnormal and Social Psychology, 73,* 256–262.

Shapiro, E.S., Browder, D.M., & D'Huyvetters, K.K. (1984). Increasing academic productivity of severely multihandicapped children with self-management: Idiosyncratic effects. *Analysis and Intervention in Developmental Disabilities, 4*(2), 171–188.

Skinner, B.F. (1979). *The role of the contrived reinforcer.* Paper presented at the 10th annual Southern California Behavior Modification Conference, Los Angeles.

Skuse, D. (1984). Extreme deprivation in early childhood—I. Diverse outcomes for three siblings from an extraordinary family. *Journal of Child Psychology and Psychiatry, 25,* 523–541.

Skuse, D. (1984). Extreme deprivation in early childhood—II. Theoretical issues and a comparative review. *Journal of Child Psychology and Psychiatry, 25,* 543–572.

Spradlin, J.E., & Siegel, G.M. (1982). Language training in natural and clinical environments. *Journal of Speech and Hearing Disorders, 47,* 2–6.

Stokes, T.F., & Baer, D.M. (1977). An implicit technology of generalization. *Journal of Applied Behavior Analysis, 10,* 347–367.

Toscher, M., & Rupp, R. (1974). The psychological implications of deafness: The human factor. *Michigan Speech and Hearing Association Journal, 10,* 60–74.

Valverde, R. (1967). Apical dendritic spines of the visual cortex and light deprivation in the mouse. *Experimental Brain Research, 3,* 337–352.

Valverde, R. (1971). Rate and extent of recovery from dark rearing in the visual cortex of the mouse. *Brain Research, 33,* 1–11.

Walk, R.D., & Gibson, E.J. (1961). A comparative and analytical study of visual depth perception. *Psychological Monographs, 75,* 1–44.

Wetherby, A.M., Koegel, R.L., & Mendel, M. (1981). Central auditory nervous system dysfunction in echolalic autistic individuals. *Journal of Speech and Hearing Research, 24,* 420–429.

Wiesel, T.N., & Hubel, D.H. (1965). Comparison of the effects of unilateral and bilateral eye closure on cortical unit responses in kittens. *Journal of Neurophysiology, 28,* 1029–1040.

Williams, J.A., Koegel, R.L., & Egel, A.L. (1981). Response-reinforcer relationships and improved learning in autistic children. *Journal of Applied Behavior Analysis, 14,* 53–60.

Wing, D.M., & Heimgartner, L.M. (1973). Articulation carryover procedure implemented by parents. *Language, Speech, and Hearing Services in Schools, 4,* 182–189.

Zubek, J.P. (1969). *Sensory deprivation: Fifteen years of research.* New York: Appleton-Century-Crofts.

Chapter 4

Research on Community Intensive Instruction as a Model for Building Functional, Generalized Skills

Wayne Sailor, Lori Goetz, Jacki Anderson, Pam Hunt, and Kathy Gee

The kind of social validity that is necessary to social survival and dissemination needs analysis and measurement, and its measurement techniques need constant developmental research and constant quality control. It is easy to create an apparent social validity that in fact masks an irritated discontent on the part of too many members of the supposedly benefitted social groups. We need to understand far better at the present how to determine the validity of our current social validity measurements, just because too many false positives in this realm can end the entire adventure for a long time. (Baer, 1986, p. 146)

Donald Baer (1986) thus admonishes his colleagues to supply more than anecdotes and good intentions in establishing recent innovations in special education as socially valid.

Certainly Baer is correct in this position. Our concern as educators with ethical standards and quality of life issues has of late run far afield of our data

This research was supported by U.S. Department of Education Grant and Contract Nos. G008430094 and 300-82-0365. No official endorsement by the department should be inferred.

base. The changes that have occurred in special education just since 1978 are nothing short of revolutionary. In programs for students with severe disabilities alone, teaching materials have become obsolete even before they have reached the market. Whole assessment systems that were developed in recent years with large infusions of federal development money, for example, have gone unused because of the shift from norm-referenced to criterion-referenced assessment models (Gentry & Haring, 1976).

In this chapter the authors argue that generalization and maintenance are substantively anchored, as outcomes, in societal-contextual relevance. *This statement means that motivation is indeed an issue apart from situational contingencies of reinforcement* (cf. Goetz, Schuler, & Sailor, 1983). The term *"context relevance"* is used here as a take-off point for examining sources of motivation that seem to occur under certain conditions of instruction and performance.

Context relevance is easily acceptable on an anecdotal basis. Under education's older model, learners were passive recipients of academic exercises to improve their competence. They were continually tested, and when they were right, they were rewarded, usually with something unrelated to the stimulus supplied in the test situation. Sufficiently powerful (but unrelated) reinforcers would increase proficiency, but that proficiency was *situationally bound* (Warren, Rogers-Warren, Baer, & Guess, 1980). Under the model prevalent today, learners are active participants in the learning situation. The accomplishment of relevant, *personal* objectives in a social transaction (however primitive at first) seems to draw performances from the learner, which then recur in appropriate future social contexts. According to this model, learning seems to progress with fewer training trials (or opportunities to initiate or respond) than has typically been the case, and often the contextual reinforcers are more subtle, seemingly less powerful than the sweets and lavish praise that frequently greeted our students' earlier efforts.

Context relevance is conceived here as a microtheoretical model that, in part, predicts generalization and maintenance of newly learned skills by students with extensive and severe disabilities. Context relevance theory is made operational by the following factors:

1. A skill to be learned has immediate *utility* for the student; it either produces something useful for the student or is part of a broader skill that does so
2. A skill has *desirability* for the student; it produces something for the student that would likely be chosen by the student if an appropriate choice situation were arranged
3. A skill is acquired in a *social* context; its acquisition is the product of interactions with more than a single (care-giving) person

4. A skill is acquired in the *actual, physical contexts* in which the skill will ultimately be requested of the student
5. A skill has *practicality* for the student; the skill is likely to be needed and practiced with some reasonable frequency
6. A skill is *appropriate* to the student's age; it will facilitate the student's increasing movement into less dependent and more integrated circumstances
7. A skill is *adaptable*; its cluster of topographical boundaries are sufficiently diffuse to enable the student to respond to the needs of different stimulus configurations (situations) with appropriate adaptations, including different exemplars of materials where needed

Consider, for example, "integrated" therapy services as a case in point for students with severe disabilities in public education programs. Language therapy has historically taken place in a pull-out fashion. A child would be removed from his or her class by the therapist, would be taken to a small room down the hall, and would be drilled with repeated trials on linguistic content that was often arbitrary and *irrelevant* for that child's future functioning in age-appropriate, normal, environmental settings. Kent-Udolf and Sherman (1983), Nietupski, Schutz, and Ockwood (1980), Lyon and Lyon (1980), and Sailor and Guess (1983), among others, have presented the rationale for the more contextually relevant model. Under such a model, teachers work together with both language therapists and parents in a consultative relationship that examines the students' communicative needs in a variety of natural settings, including interactions with a range of different individuals in multiple environments. The social context is the focus of communicative intent, and so should provide the crucible for forging initial linguistic competence.

This chapter examines selected, current research into the establishment of functional, generalized skills in students with severe disabilities as these studies relate to context relevance. First the chapter examines the components of the instructional model—which the authors have elsewhere labeled "Integrated Community Intensive Instruction" (Sailor et al., 1986)—that, in the authors' view, contribute directly to issues of generalization and maintenance. Next, the ingredients of the theoretical model described here as context relevant are delineated. Finally, the chapter examines a series of studies that lends support to the analysis of generalization and maintenance afforded by context relevance theory.

INTEGRATED, COMMUNITY INTENSIVE INSTRUCTION

The integrated community intensive instructional model is based on the assumption that all individuals, including those with the most severe disabilities, should be taught the skills to enable them to live, work, and recreate successfully in integrated environmental settings. According to this assumption, the purpose of education is thus to ensure normalized community participation by providing systematic instruction in skills essential to success within the social and environmental contexts in which those skills ultimately will be used by the student. Education should then result in life-style changes that can only occur if functional skills generalize and are maintained. To achieve this level of change, instruction within our model takes place across three broad types of environmental settings: the classroom, integrated school settings outside the classroom, and the community at large.

The authors believe that with only minor differences in technique of application, the foregoing remarks also pertain to the educational programs that have been variously described as "the community classroom" (Gaylord-Ross, Forte, & Gaylord-Ross, in press); "community-based instruction" (Baumgart & VanWallaghem, 1986; Beebe & Karan, 1986; Meyer & Evans, 1986; Vogelsberg, Ashe, & Williams, 1986); "community-referenced instruction" (Horner & McDonald, 1982; Snell & Browder, 1986); "community instruction" (Ford & Mirenda, 1984); and "community-based training station" (Stainback, Stainback, Nietupski, & Hamre-Nietupski, 1986).

This chapter is concerned with the population of developmentally disabled persons who experience the most significant delays and who may have many disabilities in addition to retardation. In special education, the population is usually described as "severely handicapped." As with any attempt to delimit a population on the basis of characteristics, there is a range and diversity in such a group. At one end of the age-expectation-performance continuum are students and clients who have profound intellectual disabilities and who may be deaf-blind, and medically fragile, for example. This group includes most people who have been labeled autistic. At the other end of the continuum are persons who exhibit some basic expressive communication skills and who might benefit from some limited remedial academic programs, such as reading and computer use. No person would be considered so disabled as not to be included in this population, but many persons might acquire a sufficient repertoire of skills to "graduate" out of the population of interest here.

Members of this population have until relatively recently (circa 1978–1980) received educational and social services primarily under a "protectionist ethic;" that is, services were sheltered and treatment/survival oriented. In the last several years, the "independent living" ethic has become more prevalent in educational and social services and, for the population of interest here, this has meant a shift in the direction of more challenging experiences and a focus on future nonsheltered work and living options. Apart from issues of whether less protective and sheltered service delivery systems are programmatically *better* for the severely disabled population, there is nonetheless a societal drift in di-

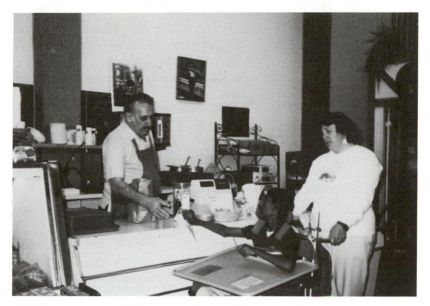

Skill instruction occurs in multiple nonschool environments as part of the community-intensive model.

rections consistent with integrated, community intensive instruction. Stronger federal enforcement of and attention to the concept of least restrictive environment (LRE) as it is embodied in PL 94-142 is a manifestation of this drift, as are many recent court decisions, such as those reviewed by Martin (1986).

Community intensive instructional methods are in their infancy. There is scant research in support of the various models that have emerged to date, yet it is clear that these models are proliferating. Much of the momentum is a logical outgrowth of the still young integration movement. The movement of students with severe disabilities from segregated school facilities to the regular public school campus, has taught us much about the relative benefits of contacts with general education peers (see Sailor, Anderson, Filler, Halvorsen, & Goetz, 1987), and a corresponding amount has been learned about the relative inappropriateness of *classrooms per se* for the education of this population, particularly in its upper age ranges.

A major issue is whether or not there is a necessary relationship between the educational concepts of integration on the one hand and community instruction on the other. As Biklen and Foster (1985) have pointed out, it is possible to "institutionalize" people in community-based programs. It is an all-too-familiar sight to see a group of young retarded adults shepherded through a park or a university campus. If simple provision of experience in community settings defined the independent variable of interest, then it is doubtful that a comparison of integrated and segregated programs would supply significant differences. What is implied here is more than simply the use of nonschool settings for instruction. Clearly, *context* must be used as an instructional tool. Specifically, the natural cues and consequences, and series of events occurring within normalized activities and environments, must provide advantageous setting events for instruction. *Context relevance,* as delineated earlier, is the underlying theoretical basis for instruction in increasingly varied school and community settings. The components of a community intensive model in this way operationalize the theory of context relevance. The next section more closely examines the elements of a community-based instructional model.

INGREDIENTS OF AN INTEGRATED COMMUNITY INTENSIVE INSTRUCTIONAL MODEL

The principal components of an integrated community intensive instructional model are:

1. A primary focus on decreasing the differences between severely disabled students and nondisabled peers by keeping activities, settings, and instructional materials age-appropriate, and by keeping a natural ratio of disabled to nondisabled persons in all instructional contexts
2. Instruction that occurs across many school and surrounding community environments and is imparted by a variety of adults and peers
3. Structured, sustained interactions among disabled and nondisabled age peers that are fostered and encouraged by teaching staff
4. Instructional technology and adaptations that are utilized such that each student participates, at least partially, in a variety of age-appropriate activities in integrated domestic, recreational, school, and vocational settings
5. Maintenance of a functional life skills curriculum focus in which all educational intervention is measured against the "criterion of ultimate functioning" or the degree to which the curriculum enhances the ability of a student to perform as independently as possible in current and subsequent natural environments (cf. L. Brown, Nietupski, & Hamre-Nietupski, 1976)
6. An instructional model wherein teaching occurs as much as possible in the context in which the taught skills will ultimately be performed, in order to capitalize on naturally occurring stimuli, routines, and motivational factors
7. An integrated therapy model in which teachers, parents, and therapists

work together to determine basic skill needs and to provide appropriate intervention in natural contexts

8. A commitment to the likelihood of a nonsheltered future that stresses work and maximally independent living circumstances

The amount of instructional time spent in each of the three types of environmental settings (classroom, nonclassroom within school, and community) varies by the student's chronological age. The general trend is to provide more instruction within the school setting during the younger ages, with a gradual increase in time spent in the community throughout the middle and high school years. Ideally, by graduation the most severely disabled student is spending all of his or her school time outside of the classroom. During this time the student is engaged primarily in work and community living skill instruction so as to facilitate a smooth transition to the postschool world of work while continuing to have frequent, sustained social contacts in integrated age-appropriate situations. Figure 1 presents proposed allotments of time for various settings

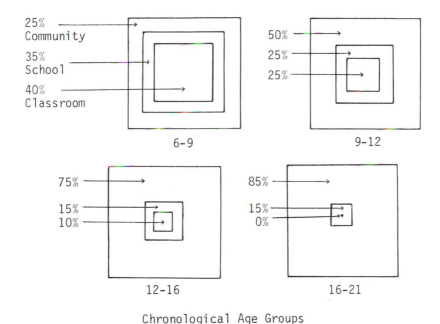

Chronological Age Groups

Figure 1.   Proposed proportional time of instruction in classroom, nonclassroom within the school, and community settings. (Reprinted with permission from Sailor, W., Halvorsen, A., Anderson, J., Goetz, L., Gee, K., Doering, K., & Hunt, P. [1986]. Community intensive instruction. In R.H. Horner, L.H. Meyer, & H.D. Fredericks [Eds.], *Education of learners with severe handicaps: Exemplary service strategies* [p. 253]. Baltimore: Paul H. Brookes Publishing Co.)

during a typical school day for various age levels, as originally recommended by Sailor et al. (1986).

More specifically, for the youngest groups, preschool and kindergarten, *mainstreaming* seems to represent the prevalent service trend in accordance with the model. Students with severe disabilities are increasingly spending most of their school time in the regular classroom in a combination special education/regular education team teaching situation. Preschool severely disabled children similarly are increasingly integrated with regular day care providers.

As the grade ladder begins for the early elementary programs, however, the service picture shifts to less time spent in the classroom and more time spent in nonclassroom school environments and in the community at large. Classroom time is increasingly likely, beginning with first grade equivalency, to be special education and not the regular classroom. As a child's developmental delays become increasingly reflected in his or her lack of reading and math ability, for example, the relevance of the regular class environment for his or her program objectives decreases substantially. At this early point, functional life skills, such as those depicted in Table 1, begin to supplement the academic curriculum focus that typifies grade one.

Table 1 presents a curriculum model, adapted from Sailor and Guess (1983), which considers a range of functional life skills, likely to be high-priority instructional objectives for students with severe disabilities, in the context of various environmental domains where increased functional skill proficiency is a high priority.

In the years up to age 12, the student is increasingly receiving instruction in nonclassroom school environments (i.e., the cafeteria, library, hallways, bathrooms, playground, etc.) and in community environments, with as much contact as possible with same-age, non–developmentally disabled peers. The instructional experiences for many such students will require physical assistance and adaptations. Participation in the regular education classroom continues on a decreased level with emphasis on nonacademic periods, such as art, music, and physical education.

At age 12, *vocational* planning and skill development begin, and community instruction starts occupying a majority of the school hours available for instruction. Finally, as the student reaches the age of transition from school to work, at about age 18, relatively little can be delivered in the classroom context that is relevant. The student's educational objectives are strongly focused on preparation for a vocational placement, for community mobility and utilization, and for semi-independent living. At this time, intensive planning occurs regarding the *transition* from the world of school to the world of work and adult services. Transition teams are beginning to be formed with representation from

Table 1. Priority matrix of functional skills

Environmental domains

Critical functions	School	Vocational	Domestic	Recreation/leisure	Community
Eating					
Toileting					
Mobility					
Expressive communication					
Receptive communication					
Horizontal social interactions					
Hygiene/ appearance					
Emergency/ safety skills					
Critical academic skills					

Adapted from Sailor and Guess (1983). *Severely handicapped students: An instructional design.* Boston: Houghton Mifflin.

school, family, and adult agencies, and plans are developed to ensure the necessary resources and support for the student to graduate to integrated work, living, and recreational settings.

Table 2 summarizes the average proportion of time spent in three instructional settings in classrooms implementing the community intensive instructional model in the San Francisco Bay area. These data are the result of direct observations in 14 Bay area classrooms (Anderson, 1984). Each age level represents classrooms serving the ranges of disabilities found in the "severely handicapped" category. As Tables 1 and 2 reveal, Bay area classrooms are not yet sufficiently developed to approximate the proportion of community-based instruction recommended by Sailor et al. (1986). Current data indicate about a 5%–9% growth per year in the proportion of community instruction due to increased development of new community instructional sites. Other factors influencing the ratio of classroom to nonclassroom and community instruction include staff ratios, homogeneous groupings of students, staff training, district policy, and transportation. Readers interested in descriptive applications of community intensive programs and their various staffing and implementation considerations are referred to Baumgart and VanWallaghem (1986), Hanson (1984), Sailor et al. (1986), Sailor and Guess (1983), and Stainback et al. (1986).

BASIS OF SUPPORT FOR COMMUNITY INTENSIVE INSTRUCTION

Since the basis for interest in the community intensive instructional model as a useful one for this population is both theoretical and philosophical, the review of the meager amount of literature available must also come from questions generated from both a research base and a philosophical/curriculum trend base.

The issues addressed in the available research literature cover a similar

Table 2. Proportion of time spent by students in various instructional settings in San Francisco Bay area classrooms implementing the community intensive instructional model

| | Percentage of school day in | | |
Population age	Classroom	Nonclassroom school	Community
4–7	40	56	4
8–11	30	44.8	25.2
12–15	31	30	39
16–22	19	23	53

Data from Anderson (1984).

broad base. Some are concerned with instructional variables (i.e., acquisition, generalization, and maintenance); others with the logistical issues of implementing instruction within the community at large, and still others with the technology itself (i.e., strategies for ecological inventories).

There is little evidence directly comparing the outcomes of community intensive intervention with outcomes of classroom-based intervention in segregated settings. There is, however, a growing body of information documenting the acquisition of specific skills as a function of training in natural environments. This training includes shopping in supermarkets (Ford, 1983), purchasing coffee in sit-down restaurants (Storey, Bates, & Hanson, 1984), social interaction in work break rooms (Breen, Haring, Pitts-Conway, & Gaylord-Ross, 1985), playing pinball machines in a public recreation center (Hill, Wehman, & Horst, 1982), playing miniature golf in a local "Putt Putt" center (Banks & Averno, 1986), conducting self-care activities in group home settings (Freagon & Rotatori, 1982), and practicing conversation skills in high school social settings (Hunt, Alwell, & Goetz, 1986).

Various logistical problems are discussed in Fimian (1984), Sailor et al. (1986), and Hamre-Nietupski, Nietupski, Bates, and Maurer (1982), and solutions to some of the logistical problems have begun to appear in recent reports. Chin-Perez et al. (1986), for example, reported a mixed community-academic instructional model that works well for heterogeneous groupings of students with disabilities at the secondary program level. Baumgart and VanWallaghem (1986) provided an analysis of eight staffing strategies that can be employed to carry out community intensive instruction, but, again, this analysis appears oriented to the higher-functioning student who can benefit both from remedial academic instruction in the classroom and from community-based instruction. The authors concluded, for example, that

> . . . the addition of community-based instruction should assist professionals in selecting the functional skills a student will learn in school to enhance performance in nonschool environments. A staffing strategy should be selected that not only allows the initial implementation of community-based instruction, but also maximizes coordination between school and nonschool instruction. (p. 101)

Snell and Browder (1986) recently provided an excellent review of research on the *technology* of community intensive instruction. Their review examined relevant research into environmental assessment approaches, including "ecological inventories" and the like; the process of task analyzing community instructional objectives; trial sequencing and stimulus control techniques; operant instructional applications to behavior management in community settings; data collection in the community; and a sample of reports of successful applications of community intensive instructional tactics across a wide variety of skill areas.

While considerable evidence exists concerning instructional, logistical, and technological variables in a community intensive model, a number of issues remain unresolved. One area of concern relates to the efficacy of a community intensive instructional model for *all* persons included in the broad category of persons with severe disabilities. The pros and cons of these trends in education were recently reviewed by F. Brown, Helmstetter, and Guess (1986), who concluded that there is virtually no empirical support for current best practices (including integrated, community intensive instruction) with the most profoundly disabled segment of the population we have been describing as "students with severe disabilities." Tawney and Demchack (1984) have similarly raised a question about the interpretation of efficacy studies within so broad and heterogeneous a group as are being addressed here. Finally, Brown et al. (1986) surveyed 236 research articles across five journals and concluded that only 1% were directed specifically at students with profound disabilities.

The authors' own anecdotal analysis suggests a tripartite problem. The most profoundly disabled members of the spectrum are being dutifully exposed to community settings, are being wheeled into supermarkets, transported on city buses, and so on, but with little evidence that much of the effort is directly beneficial. On the other hand, the curricular predecessor to this model— nonuseful, age-inappropriate activities in a classroom located in a segregated facility—produced no evidence of efficacy either, and seemed to be associated with much less instructor enthusiasm.

In the middle of the continuum is a majority of the "severe disability" population, who are well below grade level academically by the time they reach upper elementary school-age equivalency, and who yet acquire skills at a reasonable pace under community-based instructional conditions. At the top end of the spectrum are students who approach grade level in some areas, so that they require constant decision points concerning their participation in academic and remedial academic classroom work relative to the amount of time they would spend in community intensive instruction.

Empirical analysis of community intensive instruction will no doubt continue to be forthcoming. Context relevance theory, as discussed next, may prove a potential framework for such analyses.

BASIS OF SUPPORT FOR CONTEXT RELEVANCE THEORY

Context relevance theory, as delineated earlier, is intended to extend knowledge about how to produce acquisition of new skills by students with severe disabilities and, more importantly for this chapter, about how to increase generalization and maintenance of these new skills. It is not suggested as a theory of generalization per se. Rather, information derived from studies of context relevance is likely to enhance the production of generalization, when specific operations from the theory are applied in an instructional context. Context relevance is in large measure a theory of *motivation*. It suggests that certain arrangements of the socioenvironmental context of instruction will maximize the severely disabled student's motivation and ability to acquire and generalize a new skill. Thus, stated simply, *context relevance is an organized system of predicted outcomes when relevant personal objectives are accomplished in a normal social context.*

At present, context theory encompasses four general hypotheses, each of which predicts specific outcomes under certain environmental arrangements of community intensive instruction. Each of these general hypotheses provides a particular focus for organizing research relative to integrated, community intensive instruction, and each offers an interpretive framework for various ongoing and completed studies. The general hypotheses are:

1. Skill acquisition and skill generalization by students with severe disabilities are partially a function of the extent to which instruction occurs in a context of *reciprocal horizontal interactions*.
2. Skill acquisition and generalization are enhanced by employment of the principle of *functional competence*.
3. Skill acquisition and generalization are enhanced by the extent to which instruction occurs under *conditions of associated cues and effects*.
4. Skill acquisition and generalization are enhanced by the extent to which instruction is imparted through the method of *interrupted habitual chains* of behavior.

Studies Relevant to the Hypothesis of Reciprocal Horizontal Interaction

The hypothesis of enhanced motivation accruing to situations involving reciprocal horizontal (child to child) interactions is largely an outgrowth of anecdotal observations by the authors. Dramatic changes have often seemed to occur when students with severe disabilities, who were formerly segregated, were brought into a social context of intense involvement with same-age, nondisabled peers. Much of the early enthusiasm shown by special educators in response to the push for integration from Lou Brown (Brown et al., 1983) and others seemed to be corroborated by these observations. There seemed to be something magic about regular and sustained contact with nondisabled age mates that produced increased responsiveness and indications of positive affect, even in students who had been largely unresponsive in the absence of these contacts. The focus of research under this hypothesis has thus been to discover elements of the child-child interactive process that might explain increased responsiveness, and to validate the assumption that this increase would be reflected in more efficient instruction in new skill acquisition and generalization.

Much of the available research on horizontal interaction has been discussed in detail elsewhere (Sailor et al. 1987; Sailor et al., 1986); however, a number of studies merit comment. Anderson and Goetz (1983) conducted a comparative study of the nature of social interaction available in segregated versus integrated sites. Interactions were measured using the EASI (Educational Assess-

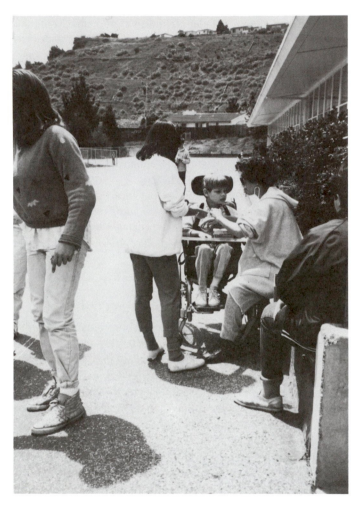

Social interactions between students appear to be an important factor in content relevance theory.

ment of Social Interaction) checklist (Goetz, Haring, & Anderson, 1983). The results indicated (perhaps obviously) that there were significantly more opportunities for interaction between severely disabled children and nondisabled children in the integrated setting. Of more importance, these researchers found that 100% of the interactions that were sampled in the segregated settings were *vertical* (from a nondisabled adult "caregiver" to a severely disabled child). In the integrated settings, 89% of the total interactions were *horizontal* (child to child), and only 11% were vertical "caregiver" interactions.

Goldstein and Wickstrom (1986) taught nondisabled children specific strategies to promote *communicative* interactions on the part of their preschool disabled classmates. The intervention resulted in increased rates of communicative interactions as well as generalizations, particularly in the incidence of "on topic" responding to initiations from the nondisabled children. The authors expressed the conclusion that "peers who act as intervention agents in one setting or activity will also share in many other activities with the handicapped child, and can thus serve as common stimuli for interactive behavior in untrained settings" (p. 214).

Murata (1984) conducted a study to evaluate a role-playing procedure for training nondisabled peers to play age-appropriate games with severely disabled students. Her dependent variable was changes in the severely disabled students' social interaction behaviors. A multiple baseline design revealed significant positive changes across three students as an outcome of the peer training procedure.

Lord and Hopkins (1986) reported a study in which they examined the social behavior of children with autism in interactive dyads with both same-age (10–12 years old) and younger (5–6 years old) nondisabled peers. In this study, the nondisabled children were not specifically trained in ways to interact with the autistic children, yet the results indicated that when opportunities to spontaneously interact in dyads were presented, the autistic children not only spontaneously interacted, as measured by several indices, but they generalized interactive skills to still other nondisabled peers. The effects were stronger with the same-age peer dyads.

Finally, several recent studies have examined benefits to disabled children from structured efforts to improve interactions with their nondisabled *siblings*. Powell, Salzberg, Rule, Levy, and Itzkowitz (1983) trained parents to engage in particular strategies to promote more functional and effective interactions between their disabled children and those children's nondisabled siblings. Sustained, generalized improvement in interactions was associated with parents' acquisition of the trained skills.

James and Egel (1986) evaluated a direct prompt training strategy to increase reciprocal interactions between and, by generalization, among siblings.

Using a multiple baseline design across three pairs of siblings, the authors' training procedures, which consisted of direct prompting and modeling techniques, resulted in increased reciprocal interactions, including expanded levels of imitations by the disabled preschool-aged children, and generalization of improved interaction skills to other play groups. The changes in interactive behavior were further shown to maintain themselves at least 6 months after intervention.

Brinker's (1985) large sample studies on integration provide still further support for the importance of horizontal interactions. The degree of integration measured in this study was the rate per minute of social bids that severely disabled students directed toward nondisabled students in the environment. In this sample, 245 students with severe disabilities of all school ages were observed over eight 10-minute observation periods scheduled throughout the school year. The most significant proportion of the total variance in this multiple regression study that predicted the degree of integration was the amount of social behavior that was directed toward the students with severe disabilities. The authors concluded that nondisabled, same-age peers are the key to successful integration efforts.

What, of applied significance, can be attributed to the outcomes of the research to date on the nature and efficacy of horizontal social interactions? There is a growing body of evidence that students with severe disabilities are indeed motivated to interact with their nondisabled age mates and that these interactions facilitate acquisition and generalization of a range of contextually relevant skills. The evidence also suggests that horizontal relationships can and should be directly facilitated by teaching staff, if such relationships are not specifically trained. Toward this end, Fowler, in Chapter 7 of this book, provides an extended analysis of procedures for facilitating peer-peer interactions and the differential effects of various types of peer-peer relationships (e.g., friend, tutor, guide).

Much research remains to be done to shed light on the elements of horizontal relationships that most directly benefit instructional goals and objects. Research is needed on the differential nature of various styles of horizontal interactions, such as peer tutorials, compared to spontaneous, nontutorial friendship relationships (cf. Haring, Breen, Pitts-Conway, Lee, & Gaylord-Ross, 1984; Murata, 1984; Selby, 1985; Smith, 1984; Voeltz, 1980; 1982).

The point of this hypothesis is that a part of context relevance (in this case the relevance of the *social* context) that enhances instruction in natural community environments accrues to the presence of reciprocal interactive relationships among students with severe disabilities and their nondisabled age mates. The question for the future is how to apply more effectively this knowledge to increase the motivation of these students to acquire socially beneficial skills.

Studies Relevant to the
Hypothesis of Functional Competence

The hypothesis of functional competence (Goetz, Schuler, & Sailor, 1979, 1981, 1983) argues that various actions that result in positive changes in the relationships between a person with severe disabilities and his or her environment will generate a motivational value that is *in addition* to the value of the act as measured by the power of the immediate reinforcer generated by the act. This additional motivation can help to generate efforts in new situations by building enhanced resistance to extinction in the context of initial skill-building activities across a range of situations. The standard societal maxim for this principle in everyday life is "nothing succeeds like success." It has close conceptual ties to the theory of "effectance motivation" espoused by R.W. White (1959). White's idea was that people learning new tasks in a series would be highly motivated by early successes in the series and that this motivation would accumulate over the series to a point where it would directly affect success on later tasks in the series. Effectance motivation was most concerned with the desire to *cause an event to occur.* This is in contrast to the desire to simply *have* the resulting event occur. The motivation lies in the act of having *caused* or *affected* the event versus the mere occurrence of the event itself. Functional competence, in practice, produces activity on the part of a student that can appear to an observor that the student is "exhilarated" from a chain of early successes and is "building up steam" to try new challenges. Koegel and Koegel, in Chapter 3, describe this phenomenon in terms of building generalized "responsivity" with children who previously acted uninterested in this environment. These are anecdotal descriptions familiar to most practicing teachers.

Motivation and competence have been closely linked by many educators and psychologists. Hrncir, Speller, and West (1985) concluded that it is difficult to tease apart competence and motivation. The more proficient children are at mastering tasks on their own, the more inclined they might be to maximize their potentials in testing and learning situations. Motti, Cicchetti, and Stroufe (1983) also emphasized the elusive and highly relative contributions of intellectual competence on the one hand, and motivation on the other, in the development of young children.

Brinker and Lewis (1982a), in a review of the reasons that infants with developmental disabilities are at risk for deprivation of contingent experiences, narrowed the many causes to two main factors: 1) Many of the conditions that cause developmental handicaps have a considerable motor component. As a result, the infant may not be able to *engage the environment* because he or she lacks the necessary movements to do so; and 2) Often parents are counseled to lower their expectations, which affects how they interact with their child.

Brinker and Lewis (1982b) suggested that both causes lead to a devastating developmental problem: a motivational deficit. The infant or child may begin to lose interest in a world over which he or she cannot exert control.

Predictability and control over environmental events has also been linked to the literature on "learned helplessness" (Peterson & Seligman, 1983). Briefly, learned helplessness is a condition in which the person exhibits a lack of motivation and nonresponsiveness. Diminished behavioral initiative and emotional disturbance is a result of the extent to which a person experiences uncontrollable events, positive or negative. Seligman asserts that the experience of controllable events produces a sense of mastery and a resistance to depression. (See Koegel and Koegel, Chapter 3, for a review of the "learned helplessness" literature.)

In a review of the literature on noncontingent stimulation, both positive and negative, Watson (1977) concluded that the eventual failure to initiate instrumental activity on the part of a person appears to be a consequence of his experiencing major sequences of events that are not *dependent* on his behavior. In a more recent study, Watson, Hayes, & Vietze (1982) demonstrated an unexpected decline in an infant's response level when the reinforcing event was *lengthened*, giving the infant fewer opportunities to *act* but more *reinforcement*. Their conclusion was that the infant's goal was to exert *control*, and that the infant preferred shorter durations of reinforcement with more chances to affect outcomes versus lengthened reinforcement and fewer opportunities to assert control.

Following several studies with infants, Ramey and Finkelstein (1978) stated that one variable related to competence and motivation is the child's attentional processes. They suggested that noncontingent stimulation causes the child to attend more to the stimulus than to his or her own behavior, and that experiences of contingent stimulation create a better balance of attention to stimuli as well as to "own actions." They hypothesized that when the child attends to his or her own *actions* as well as to the *stimulus*, the child is more likely to become aware of his ability to control the events.

The functional competence hypothesis suggests that the experience of mastery or competence over functional, natural events teaches the student to more aptly discriminate the cues for required action. Herrnstein (1970), for example, discovered that a nonlinear relationship exists between ongoing reinforcement and behavioral performance in laboratory animals, a relationship that has come to be known as "Herrnstein's hyperbola." McDowell (1982) sought an explanation for this relationship based on observations of clients in psychotherapy. The issue in these studies was how to account for the evidence of increased motivation resulting from a series of successes that could not be explained by an aggregate of the identified reinforcers in these situations. The task for the researcher today is to carefully delineate and harness the specific components of the functional competence effect that can be translated into beneficial teaching practices.

Perhaps the most direct evidence for a functional competence effect of the "learning to learn" variety with disabled children as subjects was provided in a study by Farb and Throne (1978). The investigators improved the performance of young children with Down syndrome on the Digit Span subtest of the *Wechsler Intelligence Scale for Children* (Wechsler, 1974). In the context of a multiple baseline design across digit series of increasing length, which included probes for still other untrained subtest items, the study revealed a spread of effect from training on items of one subtest to other nontrained items within the subtest, and to items from other subtests *that bore no identifiable relationships to the subtest (Digit Span) being trained,* other than the unified construct of "intelligence" that underlies all of the subtests of the intelligence test.

In another fascinating study, Halvorsen (1983) successfully improved the performance of three severely disabled students across subtests on the Uzgiris-Hunt *Ordinal Scales of Psychological Development* (Uzgiris & Hunt, 1975) through the use of systematic instructional techniques to facilitate "stage six" behavior on the first subscale: Visual Pursuit and Object Permanence. Using a multiple baseline design across three preferred, age-appropriate objects for each student with concurrent generalization probes, Halvorsen demonstrated acquisition of the highest possible object permanence response on the subscale (Step 15: location of object following three "invisible" displacements) by three of four students, with generalization of the response across novel nontrained objects by two of the participants. In addition, overall score gains on the Uzgiris-Hunt scales ranged from 7 to 13 steps between pre- and posttests. A return to baseline procedures as well as a third Uzgiris-Hunt assessment occurred in the maintenance phase, 1 month after the conclusion of the intervention. Results indicated that, on the Object Permanence subscale, students maintained gains of 1 to 5 steps over their pretest scores. The data indicate that those students who demonstrated the greatest direct benefit from the specific object permanence training also showed the greatest gain across the Uzgiris-Hunt subscales of Means, Vocal Imitation, Gestural Imitation, Operational Causality, and Spatiality.

For example, Student 1, who achieved the highest acquisition and generalization scores across objects during intervention, also showed concurrent gains across subscales, resulting in an overall posttest score 13 steps above pretest, with maintenance of 11 of these steps. The remaining Students 2 and 4, who had demonstrated acquisition and some generalization of the object permanence response, showed concurrent gains across all subscales with the following exceptions: Operational Causality for Student 2, who was at the top step of this scale in the pretest; Spatiality, for which Student 2 maintained his pretest score of 10 out of 11 steps, and Vocal Initiation, in which Student 4 maintained her pretest score. These two participants maintained overall gains of five and eight steps, respectively, above their total pretest scores. These gains are summarized in Table 3.

Again, the spread of effect apparent from these data is difficult to interpret in a context of linear, summated reinforcement for discrete responses during training on one of the six subscales.

The functional competence position also argues that early *communicative* acts that elicit immediate, positive changes in the relationships between the person with severe disabilities and his or her environment will generate a motivational value that transcends the immediate value of the act as measured by the power of the immediate reinforcer produced by the act. The additional motivation accruing to these communicative acts will help to generate new and expanded linguistic efforts by facilitating communicative efforts in new situations. The functional competence model presents some specific guidelines for the development of an initial lexicon in severely disabled students, which can only be adequately programmed in community intensive instructional programs (Goetz, Schuler, & Sailor, 1983).

Much of the relevant research on this issue has been done in conjunction with studies of the acquisition of language by children with autism and with severe retardation. Guess, Sailor, and Baer (1974), for example, first argued that efforts to teach functional speech and language to children with severe disabilities should concentrate on building *expressive* repertoires before teaching *receptive* language, in order to capitalize on the motivating power of the instrumental function of language.

Stafford, Sundberg, and Braam (1978), for example, compared the instrumental (active environmental change) function of language with the informational function (descriptive) in teaching an 11-year-old retarded male expressive signing responses. In the instrumental condition, a reinforcement item was

Table 3. Pretest, posttest, and maintenance scores on the Uzgiris and Hunt Ordinal Scales of Psychological Development

Student	Total scores on six subscales (55 total points possible)		
	Pretest	Posttest	Maintenance
1	41	54	52
2	43	50	48
3	35	42	39
4	39	50	47

Data from Halvorsen (1983).

placed in the location described by the response prior to asking the question, "Where?" In the descriptive condition, the teacher merely pointed to an empty location and asked, "Where?" In both conditions, reinforcement was randomly selected from among four predetermined reinforcers. Thus, in the instrumental condition, a correct response functioned as a successful request for a specific item, while in the informational condition, the function of the response was descriptive in nature and not directly related to the reinforcement received. The results suggested that teaching a communication behavior that provides direct control over specific environmental events was a superior strategy to teaching a purely informational response when other motivational factors were controlled. Similarly, Janssen and Guess (1978) compared acquisition of object discrimination skills in four profoundly retarded subjects. In one condition, a discrimination was taught using typical edible reinforcers. In the other condition, a correct response led to an opportunity to physically manipulate the discriminated object. The subjects performed significantly better in the latter condition.

Finally, Goetz (1981) controlled motivational factors across conditions in a receptive language labeling study with severely disabled students. In a functional manipulation condition, correct labeling responses resulted in tangible reinforcement and concurrent training in functional use of the object that had been named (i.e., stapling with a stapler). In an alternate condition, correct responses resulted in tangible reinforcement and the opportunity to manipulate the item, but no direct instruction in purposeful use of the item was provided. Conditions were counterbalanced for order across four students. Results for two of the students are presented in Figure 2. These results suggest more rapid acquisition (as reflected by steeper slope lines) for the functional manipulation condition, in which correct responses were associated with the opportunity to experience motoric competence with the stimulus item.

In a series of studies designed to teach children to use their residual vision in order to control visual-motor actions (Gee & Goetz, 1985; Goetz & Gee, 1987), it was repeatedly found that so long as the use of visual fixation brought students success in situations involving motor actions, such as fixating while inserting a bubble wand into a jar of bubbles, the acquisition and maintenance of vision use remained high. When the student, however, used his or her vision but was still unable to successfully complete the motor act, vision use decreased in those situations, while continuing in situations in which vision use facilitated successful task performance. Thus, vision use that resulted in active environmental control of events was selectively learned and maintained.

These findings support the hypothesis of functional competence expressed as a facilitation of learning by active participation. The findings have significance for the development of teaching methods to instill generalization and maintenance. They would, for example, suggest using *contextual prompts* over

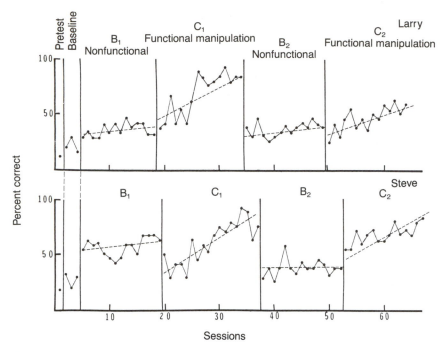

Figure 2. Percentage of correct trials per session for two students. ●—● indicates perfor-mance data for two students in alternating conditions. ---- indicates trend lines. (Reprinted with permission from Goetz, L. [1981]. *Effects of functional object use on acquisition of receptive labeling skills: An experimental analysis of semantic development in severely handicapped learners.* Unpublished doctoral dissertation, University of California at Berkeley and San Francisco State University.)

verbal and physical prompting procedures wherever possible. Again, the litera-ture on "learned helplessness" reviewed by Koegel and Koegel (Chapter 3) is relevant in this context. Just as the "therapy" for the experimental dogs that had displayed a kind of learned helplessness was to facilitate their opportunities to make an *instrumental* response to the aversive stimulus, efforts by teachers to create opportunities for students to *initiate* actions designed to acquire new skills should facilitate generalized learning.

The implications of findings such as these for application by teachers, par-ticularly with respect to the establishment of generalization, have much to do with organizing instructional trials so as to *maximize early successes*. Cer-tainly the "errorless" instructional procedures demonstrated by Touchette (1971) would be called for. The practice of instructing groups of diverse skills in natural chains, such as represented by the Kansas Individualized Curriculum

Sequencing model (KICS) (Holvoet, Mulligan, Schussler, Lacy, & Guess, 1982; Sailor & Guess, 1983) would also be suggested by this analysis.

Finally, the functional competence hypothesis would predict at least a slight negative effect for the use of correction procedures. Whatever momentum accrues to the buildup of early successes in a chain would likely be extinguished with the interjection of mild verbal punishers and the requirement of repeating trials that usually constitutes a standard correction procedure. There may well, however, be cases where a correction procedure is unavoidable, such as in the negative case example procedure discussed by Albin and Horner in Chapter 5 of this book, in the context of the general-case instruction procedure. It should be noted that the functional competence hypothesis predicts an *enhancement* of generalized learning when its conditions can be fulfilled, but it is not postulated to be *necessary* for generalized learning to occur.

Studies Relevant to the
Hypothesis of Associated Cues and Effects

The associated cue and effect hypothesis can be stated as follows: *Generalized new learning will be enhanced to the extent that it occurs under conditions of maximum physical correlation among the stimuli discriminative for reinforcement, the responses to be reinforced, and the reinforcers.* The "natural cues and consequences" model proposed by Falvey, Brown, Lyon, Baumgart, and Schroeder (1980) offers teaching suggestions that are consistent with this hypothesis.

Saunders and Sailor (1979), and later Litt and Schreibman (1982), examined a *"specific reinforcer"* relationship in a discriminative learning paradigm and concluded that something extra is gained in learning efficiency when reinforcers are made specific to the stimuli and acts that produce them. For example, in the Saunders and Sailor (1979) study, subjects were better able to match names of toys to actual toys when the reinforcer for correct naming was a chance to play with the named toy. This condition was contrasted with one in which the children could play with yet another toy that had previously been determined to be of greater choice value, as a reinforcer for correct name-matching with the less desirable toys. This procedure is in contrast to the more common situation of programming ubiquitous reinforcers for various behaviors.

Similarly, Koegel and Williams (1980) tailored specific reinforcers to a series of verbal, motor, imitative, and receptive labeling acts and contrasted this relationship with a condition in which responses were reinforced with an item not specific to the responses taught. With autistic children as subjects, the results replicated the findings of the Saunders and Sailor (1979) and Litt and Schreibman (1982) efforts. In a later study, Williams, Koegel, and Egel (1981) examined three children with autism for a comparison of systematically arbitrary versus functional relationships between target behaviors and reinforcers. Using a multiple baseline design across subjects and behaviors, the results of the study indicated that functional response-reinforcer relationships produced immediate improvement in the learning of functional skills. Further, results showed that the high level of correct responding produced under this condition were maintained even when the previously ineffective arbitrary response-reinforcer conditions were reinstated. The authors interpreted the results in a context of the relevance of contextual cues. Functional response-reinforcer relationships, according to this analysis, helped to enhance the discrimination of the contingency between the reinforcers and the intended target behavior, and may therefore help to focus the autistic child's attention on relevant portions of the teaching task.

Halvorsen's study (1983), discussed earlier, also employed the use of reinforcers (food, toys) specific to the object permanence task being trained. She hypothesized that the fact that students were allowed to eat (food) or play with (toy) the object after locating it, contributed to the success of the intervention.

A number of studies growing out of the associated cues and effects hypothesis have been conducted on generalized use of residual vision and orientation and mobility instruction in natural environments (Gee & Goetz, 1985, 1986; Gee, Harrell, & Rosenberg, 1987).

Gee and Goetz (1986), for example, taught basic orientation and mobility skills to four students with severe disabilities within the context of several functional travel routes, despite evidence from the *Peabody Mobility Scale* (Harley, Wood, & Merbler, 1980) that the students failed to meet the prerequisites (e.g., concept discrimination) for such training. The students were able to generalize their new motoric mobility skills, such as trailing and turning corners, to unfamiliar routes. They also demonstrated a high level of incidental learning of the landmarks, clues, and memory tasks specific to the training routes. This research is in contrast to earlier orientation and mobility instruction models that taught skills in a sequential/prerequisite fashion, with the expectation that students with severe, multiple disabilities would be able to integrate concept lessons such as right/left, up/down into movement situations in natural community contexts similar to students whose only disability is blindness. Instead of training prerequisite skills in isolation, instruction was given using "interspersed" training trials (e.g., instruction on a few initial skills was given as the opportunity arose within the ongoing movement of the travel route, and the student was assisted on the remaining parts of the route). Instruction thus occurred within the actual travel routes, with the setting event or "chain of behaviors" providing both the natural cues and cue-specific consequences for performance of the motor skills being taught.

Similarly, Gee and Goetz (1985) and Goetz and Gee (1987) taught use of residual vision in conjunction with fine-motor behaviors (visual-motor skills) within ongoing activity routines of play, household or classroom chores, and self-care tasks. The most important component of the instructional paradigm was the highly correlated context set up for the use of vision. Completion of the task within the activity routine was made contingent upon the use of vision. Maintained visual fixation was then instructed using a form of time delay (Touchette, 1971). The method required that instruction only occur at the natural points where the visual skill was *necessary* to the continuation of the task/ play, etc. These studies suggest that by first reviewing the student's participation in activities that are age-appropriate and necessary for increased independence (i.e., community intensive instruction), the teacher is one step closer to determining the critical moments within those activities and natural settings that require the use of visual-motor skills and, thus, the points where instruction can occur effectively.

Clearly, although the available research in support of the hypothesis of correlated cues and effects is sparse, the evidence is also highly intriguing. Research on the *nature* of reinforcing relationships may ultimately rival the scope and impact of the large body of research on the *application* of reinforcers in the production of generalized and sustained skill development with severely disabled students. Studies in context relevance theory are particularly focused, for now, on the physical relationships among cues in a learning situation and on the consequences for correctly produced responses.

Studies Relevant to the Hypothesis of Interrupted Habitual Chains of Behavior

The fourth and final hypothesis leading to focused studies of context relevance is the interrupted chain effect. This notion has its roots in Spence's (1956) work on learning theory, particularly his analysis of the principle of "habit strength." By this analysis, the likelihood that an organism will perform a learned response is predictable from knowledge of the strength of the response under conditions of habitual performance. Reinforcement, by this analysis, serves to add to the strength of the habituation process. Since behavior tends to organize into chains of responses that are habitually (repeatedly) performed in the same way under similar conditions, motivation to perform *later* elements in a chain may (hypothetically) be increased by interrupting the chain at an earlier point. Since instruction in natural community environments often requires short one- or two-trial instructional efforts within a chain of ongoing behavior, this hypothesis offers potential for helping to develop a teaching technology better suited, for example, for community instruction than massed-trial, situation-bound teaching methods. Several recent studies have been undertaken to examine this hypothesis (cf. Goetz, Gee, & Sailor, 1985; Hunt, Goetz, Alwell, & Sailor, 1986).

In this instructional paradigm, "instruction occurs directly in the midst of ongoing, active behavior, and . . . reinforcement (i.e., completion of the sequence) is a predictable environmental change that is unique to each response being learned . . ." (Goetz et al., 1985, p. 22). In this study, the authors taught pictorial communicative skills to two adolescents with severe disabilities by inserting a typical operant instructional trial into the midst of such ongoing sequences of organized behavior as making toast, washing dishes, and so forth. Comparing the interrupted chain condition with an instructional condition in which the linguistic response was taught at the beginning of each chain, the results supported the interrupted chain strategy by providing evidence for a motivational "boost" related to the specific parameters of the interrupted chain procedure.

Hunt, Goetz, Alwell, and Sailor (1986) further examined the interrupted chain procedure in terms of its efficacy in producing generalized communicative behavior with severely disabled students. In this study, three elementary school–age severely disabled students were first taught communicative acts using an interrupted behavior chain strategy, and were then tested to see if the acquired acts were under the control of a set of stimuli that shared common characteristics across a variety of interrupted routine contexts. Generalization was analyzed in terms of the extent to which the trained communicative functions (e.g., requesting), response form (e.g., pointing to a picture), and picture discrimination skills (e.g., selecting the correct picture from among an array) required for selection of the appropriate content for each communication response were used within still *other* behavior chain interruption contexts (where no training had occurred). The results indicated that instruction in an interrupted chain context resulted in rapid acquisition of specific communicative acts and in generalization of communicative functions, response forms, and picture discrimination skills to novel, untrained chain interruption contexts.

SUMMARY

Context relevance theory represents an effort to integrate a number of diverse as well as divergent research outcomes, philosophical tenets, curricular practices, and anecdotal reports, all of which are reflected in a community intensive model of instruction. Some of these components, such as the role of active integration with nondisabled peers, have strong empirical support from a variety of perspectives and research methodologies. Other components, such as the concepts of functional competence and chain interruption, are closely tied to well-developed theoretical models of human learning, such as Spence's construct of the fractional anticipatory goal response (Spence, 1956). Several other components, such as those associated with the functional competence hypothesis, have been studied for several years, from a variety of theoretical perspectives, but have lacked conceptual unification. As such, context relevance theory requires a great deal of additional investigation, and will doubtless undergo further modification in accordance with empirical data. Currently, however, it does reflect an attempt to synthesize scientific and educational "best guesses" into a format that presents some clear direction for future research.

The integrated community intensive instructional model in which context relevance theory is grounded will also no doubt continue to change in response to issues of both empirical and social validity. At present, however, the parameters of the model as discussed here appear to offer promising practices that have the potential to genuinely affect the life-style of all students with severe disabilities.

REFERENCES

Anderson, J. (1984). *San Francisco school district evaluation report: Jose Ortega school study.* Unpublished manuscript, San Francisco State University, California Research Institute.

Anderson, J., & Goetz, L. (1983, November). *Social interactions between severely handicapped students and their peers: A preliminary report.* Paper presented at the annual meeting of The Association for the Severely Handicapped, San Francisco.

Baer, D. (1986). Exemplary service to what outcome? Review of *Education of learners with severe handicaps: Exemplary service strategies. Journal of The Association for Persons with Severe Handicaps, 11*(2), 145–147.

Banks, R., & Averno, A. (1986). Adapted miniature golf: A community leisure program for students with severe physical disabilities. *Journal of The Association for Persons with Severe Handicaps, 11*(3), 209–215.

Baumgart, D., & VanWallaghem, J. (1986). Staffing strategies for implementing community-based instruction. *Journal of The Association for Persons with Severe Handicaps, 11*(2), 92–102.

Beebe, P., & Karan, O. (1986). A methodology for a community-based program for adults. In R.H. Horner, L.H. Meyer, & H.D. Fredericks (Eds.), *Education of learners with severe handicaps: Exemplary service strategies* (pp. 3–28). Baltimore: Paul H. Brookes Publishing Co.

Biklen, D., & Foster, S. (1985). Principles for integrated community programming. In M. Brady & P. Gunter (Eds.), *Integrating moderately and severely handicapped learners* (pp. 16–46). Springfield, IL: Charles C Thomas.

Breen, C., Haring, T., Pitts-Conway, V., & Gaylord-Ross, R. (1985). The training and generalization of social interaction during breaktime at two job sites in the natural environment. *Journal of The Association for Persons with Severe Handicaps, 10*(1), 41–50.

Brinker, R. (1985). Interactions between severely mentally retarded students and other students in integrated and segregated public school settings. *American Journal of Mental Deficiency, 89*(6), 587–594.

Brinker, R., & Lewis, M. (1982a). Making the world work with microcomputers: A learning prosthesis for handicapped children. *Exceptional Children, 49,* 163–170.

Brinker, R., & Lewis, M. (1982b). Discovering the competent handicapped infant: A process approach to assessment and intervention. *Topics in Early Childhood Special Education, 2*(2), 1–16.

Brown, F., Helmstetter, E., & Guess, D. (1986). *Current best practices with students with profound disabilities: Are there any?* Manuscript in preparation, University of Kansas, Lawrence.

Brown, L., Ford, A., Nisbet, J., Sweet, M., Donnellan, A., & Gruenewald, L. (1983). Opportunities available when severely handicapped students attend chronological age appropriate regular schools. *Journal of The Association for the Severely Handicapped, 8,* 16–24.

Brown, L., Nietupski, J., & Hamre-Nietupski, S. (1976). The criterion of ultimate functioning and public school services for severely handicapped students. In M.A. Thomas (Ed.), *Hey, don't forget about me: Education's investment in the severely, profoundly, and multiply handicapped* (pp. 197–209). Reston, VA: Council for Exceptional Children.

Chin-Perez, G., Hartman, D., Park, H., Sacks, S., Wersching, A., & Gaylord-Ross, R. (1986). Maximizing social contact for secondary students with severe handicaps. *Journal of The Association for Persons with Severe Handicaps, 11*(2), 118–124.

Falvey, M., Brown, L., Lyon, S., Baumgart, D., & Schroeder, J. (1980). Strategies for using cues and correction procedures. In W. Sailor, B. Wilcox, & L. Brown (Eds.), *Methods of instruction for severely handicapped students* (pp. 109–133). Baltimore: Paul H. Brookes Publishing Co.

Farb, J., & Throne, J. (1978). Improving the generalized mnemonic performance of a Down's Syndrome child. *Journal of Applied Behavior Analysis, 11,* 413–420.

Fimian, M. (1984). Organizational variables related to stress and burnout in community-based programs. *Education and Training of the Mentally Retarded, 19,* 201–209.

Ford, A. (1983). *The performance of moderately and severely handicapped students in community environments as a function of the cues available and the antecedent versus consequential teaching procedures used.* Unpublished doctoral dissertation, University of Wisconsin, Department of Behavioral Disability, Madison.

Ford, A., & Mirenda, P. (1984). Community instruction: A natural cues and corrections decision model. *Journal of The Association for Persons with Severe Handicaps, 9,* 79–87.

Freagon, S., & Rotatori, A. (1982). Comparing natural and artificial environments in training self-care skills to group home residents. *Journal of The Association for the Severely Handicapped, 7*(3), 73–86.

Gaylord-Ross, C., Forte, J., & Gaylord-Ross, R. (in press). The community classroom: Technological vocational training for students with severe disabilities. *Career Development for Exceptional Individuals.*

Gee, K., & Goetz, L. (1987). *Establishing generalized use of residual vision through instruction in natural contexts.* Manuscript in preparation. San Francisco State University, Department of Special Education, San Francisco.

Gee, K., & Goetz, L. (1987). *Outcomes of instructing orientation and mobility skills across purposeful travel in natural environments.* Manuscript in preparation. San Francisco State University, Department of Special Education, San Francisco.

Gee, K., Harrell, R., & Rosenberg, R. (1987). Teaching orientation and mobility skills within and across natural opportunities for travel: A model designed for learners with multiple severe disabilities. In L. Goetz, D. Guess, & K. Stremel-Campbell (Eds.), *Innovative program design for individuals with dual sensory impairments* (pp. 127–157). Baltimore: Paul H. Brookes Publishing Co.

Gentry, D., & Haring, N.G. (1976). Essentials of performance measurement. In N. Haring & L. Brown (Eds.), *Teaching the severely handicapped* (Vol. 1) (pp. 209–236). New York: Grune & Stratton.

Goetz, L. (1981). *Effects of functional object use on acquisition of receptive labeling skills: An experimental analysis of semantic development in severely handicapped learners*. Unpublished doctoral dissertation, University of California at Berkeley and San Francisco State University.

Goetz, L., & Gee, K. (1987). Teaching visual attention in functional contexts: Acquisition, generalization, and maintenance of complex motor skills. *Journal of Vision Impairment and Blindness, 81,* 115–117.

Goetz, L., Gee, K., & Sailor, W. (1985). Using a behavior chain interrupted strategy to teach communication skills to students with severe disabilities. *Journal of The Association for Persons with Severe Handicaps, 10*(1), 21–30.

Goetz, L., Haring, T., & Anderson, J. (1983). *Educational assessment for social interaction (EASI)*. [Eric Document Reproduction Services No. ED 242 184]. San Francisco: San Francisco State University and San Francisco Unified School District.

Goetz, L., Schuler, A., & Sailor, W. (1979). Teaching functional speech to the severely handicapped: Current issues. *Journal of Autism and Developmental Disabilities, 9,* 325–343.

Goetz, L., Schuler, A., & Sailor, W. (1981). Functional competence as a factor in communication instruction. *Exceptional Education Quarterly, 2,* 51–61.

Goetz, L., Schuler, A., & Sailor, W. (1983). Motivational considerations in teaching language to severely handicapped students. In M. Hersen, V. vanHasselt, & J. Marson (Eds.), *Behavior therapy for the developmentally and physically disabled: A handbook* (pp. 57–77). New York: Academic Press.

Goldstein, H., & Wickstrom, S. (1986). Peer intervention effects on communicative interaction among handicapped and nonhandicapped preschoolers. *Journal of Applied Behavior Analysis, 19,* 209–214.

Guess, D., Sailor, W., & Baer, D. (1974). To teach language to retarded children. In R. Schiefelbusch & L. Lloyd (Eds.), *Language perspectives—Acquisition, retardation, and intervention* (pp. 529–563). Baltimore: University Park Press.

Halvorsen, A. (1983). *The facilitation of object permanence responses through behavioral techniques with severely retarded students*. Unpublished doctoral dissertation, University of California at Berkeley and San Francisco State University.

Hamre-Nietupski, S., Nietupski, J., Bates, P., & Maurer, S. (1982). Implementing a community-based educational model for moderately/severely handicapped students: Common problems and suggested solutions. *Journal of The Association for the Severely Handicapped, 7,* 38–43.

Hanson, M. (Ed.). (1984). *Atypical infant development*. Baltimore: University Park Press.

Haring, T., Breen, C., Pitts-Conway, V., Lee, M., & Gaylord-Ross, R. (1984). The effects of peer tutoring and special friend experiences on nonhandicapped adolescents. In R. Gaylord-Ross, T. Haring, C. Breen, M. Lee, V. Pitts-Conway, & B. Roger (Eds.), *The social development of handicapped children* (Monograph). San Francisco: San Francisco State University, Department of Special Education.

Harley, R., Wood, T., & Merbler, J. (1980). An orientation and mobility program for multiply impaired blind children. *Exceptional Children, 46,* 326–331.

Herrnstein, R. (1970). On the law of effect. *Journal of Experimental Analysis of Behavior, 13,* 243–266.

Hill, J., Wehman, P., & Horst, G. (1982). Toward generalization of appropriate leisure and social behavior in severely handicapped youth: Pinball machine use. *Journal of The Association for Persons with Severe Handicaps, 6*(4), 38–44.

Holvoet, J., Mulligan, M., Schussler, N., Lacy, L., & Guess, D. (1982). *The KICS model: Sequencing learning experiences for severely handicapped children and youth.* Lawrence: University of Kansas, Department of Special Education.

Horner, R., & McDonald, R. (1982). Comparison of single instance and general case instruction in teaching of a generalized vocational skill. *Journal of The Association for Persons with Severe Handicaps, 7*(3), 7–20.

Hrncir, E., Speller, G., & West, M. (1985). What are we testing? *Developmental Psychology, 21,* 226–232.

Hunt, P., Alwell, M., & Goetz, L. (1986). *Acquisition of conversation skills and the reduction of inappropriate social interaction behaviors.* Manuscript submitted for publication.

Hunt, P., Goetz, L., Alwell, M., & Sailor, W. (1986). Using an interrupted behavior chain strategy to teach generalized communication responses to students with severe disabilities. *Journal of The Association for Persons with Severe Handicaps, 11*(3), 196–204.

James, S., & Egel, A. (1986). A direct prompting strategy for increasing reciprocal interactions between handicapped and nonhandicapped siblings. *Journal of Applied Behavior Analysis, 19*(2), 173–186.

Janssen, C., & Guess, D. (1978). Use of function as a consequence in training receptive labeling to severely and profoundly retarded individuals. *AAESPH Review, 3,* 246–258.

Kent-Udolf, L., & Sherman, E. R. (1983). *Shop talk: A prevocational language program for retarded students.* Champaign, IL: Research Press.

Koegel, R., & Williams, J. (1980). Direct vs. indirect response-reinforcer relationship in teaching autistic children. *Journal of Abnormal Psychology, 8,* 537–547.

Litt, M., & Schreibman, L. (1982). Stimulus specific reinforcement in the acquisition of receptive labels by autistic children. *Journal of Analysis and Intervention in Developmental Disabilities, 1,* 171–186.

Lord, C., & Hopkins, J. (1986). The social behavior of autistic children with younger and same-age nonhandicapped peers. *Journal of Autism and Developmental Disorders, 16*(3), 249–262.

Lyon, S., & Lyon, G. (1980). Team functioning and staff development: A role release approach to providing integrated educational services for severely handicapped students. *Journal of The Association for Persons with Severe Handicaps, 5*(3), 250–263.

Martin, R. (1986). *Ending segregation of handicapped students: Taking steps toward the least restrictive environment.* Austin: Advocacy.

McDowell, J. (1982). The importance of Herrnstein's mathematical statement of the law of effect for behavior therapy. *American Psychologist, 37,* 771–779.

Meyer, L., & Evans, I. (1986). Modification of excess behavior: An adaptive and functional approach for educational contexts. In R.H. Horner, L.H. Meyer, & H.D. Fredericks (Eds.), *Education of learners with severe handicaps: Exemplary service strategies* (pp. 315–356). Baltimore: Paul H. Brookes Publishing Co.

Motti, F., Cicchetti, D., & Stroufe, L. (1983). From infant affect expression to symbolic play: The coherence of development in Down syndrome children. *Child Development, 54*(5), 1168–1175.

Murata, C. (1984). The effects of an indirect training procedure for nonhandicapped peers on interaction response class behaviors of autistic children. In R. Gaylord-Ross, T. Haring, C. Breen, M. Lee, V. Pitts-Conway, & B. Roger (Eds.), *The social development of handicapped students* (pp. 7–30). San Francisco: San Francisco State University.

Nietupski, J., Schutz, G., & Ockwood, L. (1980). The delivery of communication services to severely handicapped students: A plan for change. *Journal of The Association for the Severely Handicapped, 5*(1), 13–24.

Peterson, C., & Seligman, M. (1983). Learned helplessness and victimization. *Journal of Social Issues, 39*(2), 103–116.

Powell, T., Salzberg, C., Rule, S., Levy, S., & Itzkowitz, J. (1983). Teaching mentally retarded children to play with their siblings using parents as trainers. *Education and Treatment of Children, 6*(4), 343-362.

Ramey, C., & Finkelstein, N. (1978). Contingent stimulation and infant competence. *Journal of Pediatric Psychology, 3,* 89–967.

Sailor, W., Anderson, J., Filler, J., Halvorsen, A., & Goetz, L. (1987). *Community intensive instruction in integrated settings: Research to practice* (Monograph in preparation). San Francisco: San Francisco State University, California Research Institute.

Sailor, W., & Guess, D. (1983). *Severely handicapped students: An instructional design.* Boston: Houghton Mifflin.

Sailor, W., Halvorsen, A., Anderson, J., Goetz, L., Gee, K., Doering, K., & Hunt, P. (1986). Community intensive instruction. In R.H. Horner, L.H. Meyer, & H.D. Fredericks (Eds.), *Education of learners with severe handicaps: Exemplary service strategies* (pp. 251–288). Baltimore: Paul H. Brookes Publishing Co.

Saunders, R., & Sailor, W. (1979). A comparison of three strategies of reinforcement on two-choice learning problems with severely retarded children. *AAESPH Review, 4*(4), 323–333.

Selby, P. (1985). *A comparison of learning acquisition by teacher instruction and handicapped peer tutor instruction on leisure and gross motor skills of three mentally retarded children.* Unpublished master's thesis, San Francisco State University.

Smith, B. (1984). *Generalization of social interactions between two autistic children and their nonhandicapped peers.* Unpublished master's thesis, California State University at Hayward.

Snell, M., & Browder, D. (1986). Community-referenced instruction: Research and issues. *Journal of The Association for Persons with Severe Handicaps, 11,* 1–11.

Spence, K. (1956). *Behavior theory and condition.* New Haven, CT: Yale University Press.

Stafford, M., Sundberg, M., & Braam, S. (1978). *An experimental analysis of mands and tacts.* Paper presented at the fourth annual convention of the Midwest Association of Behavior Analysis, Chicago.

Stainback, W., Stainback, S., Nietupski, J., & Hamre-Nietupski, S. (1986). Establishing effective community-based training stations. In F.R. Rusch (Ed.), *Competitive employment issues and strategies* (pp. 103–113). Baltimore: Paul H. Brookes Publishing Co.

Storey, K., Bates, P., & Hanson, H. (1984). Acquisition and generalization of coffee purchase skills by adults with severe disabilities. *Journal of The Association for Persons with Severe Handicaps, 9*(3), 178–185.

Tawney, J., & Demchak, M. (1984). Severely retarded? Severely handicapped? Multiply handicapped? A definitional analysis. *Topics in Early Childhood Education, 4*(3), 1–18.

Touchette, P. (1971). Transfer of stimulus control: Measuring the moment of transfer. *Journal of the Experimental Analysis of Behavior, 15*, 347–354.

Uzgiris, I., & Hunt, J. McV. (1975). *Assessment in infancy: Ordinal Scales of Psychological Development*. Urbana, IL: University Press.

Voeltz, L.M. (1980). Children's attitudes toward handicapped peers. *American Journal of Mental Deficiency, 84*, 455–464.

Voeltz, L.M. (1982). Effects of structured interactions with severely handicapped peers on children's attitudes. *American Journal of Mental Deficiency, 86*, 380–390.

Vogelsberg, R., Ashe, W., & Williams, W. (1986). Community-based services in rural Vermont: Issues and recommendations. In R.H. Horner, L.H. Meyer, & H.D. Fredericks (Eds.), *Education of learners with severe handicaps: Exemplary service strategies* (pp. 29–59). Baltimore: Paul H. Brookes Publishing Co.

Warren, S., Rogers-Warren, A., Baer, D.M., & Guess, D. (1980). Assessment and facilitation of language. In W. Sailor, B. Wilcox, & L. Brown (Eds.), *Methods of instruction for severely handicapped students* (pp. 227–258). Baltimore: Paul H. Brookes Publishing Co.

Watson, J. (1977). Depression and the perception of control in early childhood. In J. Schulterbrand & A. Raskin (Eds.), *Depression in childhood: Diagnostic, treatment, and conceptual models* (pp. 123–133). New York: Raven Press.

Watson, J., Hayes, L., & Vietze, P. (1982). Response-contingent stimulation as a treatment for developmental failure in infancy. *Journal of Applied Developmental Psychology, 3*, 191–203.

Wechsler, D. (1974). *Wechsler Intelligence Scale for Children*. New York: Psychological Corporation.

White, R.W. (1959). Motivation reconsidered: The concept of competence. *Psychological Review, 66*, 297–333.

Williams, J., Koegel, R., & Egel, A. (1981). Response-reinforcer relationships and improved learning in autistic children. *Journal of Applied Behavior Analysis, 14*(1), 53–60.

Chapter 5 ─────────────────────

Generalization with Precision

Richard W. Albin and Robert H. Horner

═══

Among the most exciting recent advances in instructional technology has been the development of procedures for teaching generalized skills (Albin, McDonnell, & Wilcox, 1987; Horner, McDonnell, & Bellamy, 1986; Horner, Sprague, & Wilcox, 1982; Stokes & Baer, 1977; Stokes & Osnes, 1986). The capability now exists to teach people, including individuals with major learning difficulties, to perform adaptive skills in nontrained situations. In the search for an applied technology of generalization, however, a danger has arisen in the implicit assumptions that: 1) all generalization is good and 2) generalization is an all-or-nothing phenomenon in which any demonstration of generalization, no matter how limited, documents adequate instruction. In fact, recent advances in generalization research have expanded the level of sophistication expected from the applied technology. To produce important behavioral changes, our technology of generalization needs to do more than teach skills that are performed in some nontrained conditions. It must teach skills that are: 1) performed *across the full range* of appropriate, nontrained conditions that the learner will encounter in his or her normal daily routine and 2) *not* be performed in inappropriate conditions (Horner, Bellamy, & Colvin, 1984).

The excitement resulting from initial demonstrations of generalization success is being tempered by the recognition that the technology for teaching generalized skills will be of little value unless we can teach skills that generalize with the precision demanded by the natural environment. Efforts to teach generalized social skills, for example, often miss the mark when those skills generalize to inappropriate situations. Successful generalization of purchasing

The activity that is the subject of this report was supported in whole or in part by the U.S. Department of Education, Contract No. 300-82-0362 and Grant No. G00-85-30233. However, the opinions expressed herein do not necessarily reflect the position or policy of the U.S. Department of Education, and no official endorsement by the department should be inferred.

99

skills across different, in-school situations is encouraging, until reports come back that this skill is not performed in real stores in the community.

This chapter describes recent advances in building a generalization technology that meets the precision demands of the real world. It presents theory and applied recommendations related to the selection of optimal teaching examples, particularly negative teaching examples, for the establishment of precise generalized responding.

COMMUNITY PERFORMANCE
REQUIRES GENERALIZATION WITH PRECISION

In recent years, professional opinion has joined with legislative imperatives to create a strong emphasis on community-based services in the least restrictive environment for persons with severe disabilities. This emphasis has major implications for what and how persons with severe disabilities are taught (Albin et al., 1987; Wilcox & Bellamy, 1987). It is not sufficient to perform some adaptive behavior under contrived or simulated training conditions, or even under some static set of natural conditions. The natural community is characterized by its variability. Adaptive behaviors often are functional only when they can be performed under a variety of stimulus conditions. It is unlikely that training can be provided in all of the varied conditions that learners will face in the natural community. Practitioners need a generalization technology that meets the demands of the natural community.

One important feature of the community is that it frequently demands a high degree of precision in learner performance. For many skills and activities, it is equally important that learners know when to respond and when not to respond. Consider a student learning to cross streets; a worker learning to bus tables in a restaurant; a bus rider in a large city waiting for the correct bus at a transit station; or a grocery shopper seeking items to match a set of photographs that serve as a grocery list. For each of these tasks, success requires responding with sufficient precision to meet the exacting demands of the community. For the tasks to be truly functional, the student must be able to respond or to not respond, depending on which is appropriate, with a precision that meets community standards rather than some arbitrary criteria set by the trainer. A technology to teach skills and activities to be used in the community must produce generalized responding that meets the precision demands and performance standards of the community.

An important implication of viewing the applied problem of generalization from the perspective of establishing precision in responding is that greater attention is focused on the issue of stimulus control over generalized responding (Horner et al., 1984; Marholin & Touchette, 1979). Stimulus control refers to a functional relationship between the presentation of an antecedent stimulus and change in the probability of a response (Terrace, 1966). The applied problem of generalization involves bringing adaptive skills and behaviors under the control of appropriate, relevant stimuli. Such a framework highlights two basic characteristics of generalization with precision in the community: 1) correct responding occurs across all nontrained conditions in which the relevant, controlling stimuli are present, not just in some limited number of nontrained conditions and 2) responding does not occur in inappropriate conditions in which relevant, controlling stimuli are not present.

Although the principle of stimulus control serves as a basis for much of our existing behavioral technology (Bellamy, Horner, & Inman, 1979), its role in solving the applied problem of generalization is not as well delineated. If referred to in such contexts at all, the tendency is to view stimulus control only as a part of some strategies for establishing generalized responding. Stokes and Osnes (1986), for example, touch briefly on the role played by stimulus control in generalization strategies, based on the underlying tactic that they term "incorporate functional mediators." More prevalent are discussions of tactics such as "train diversely (or loosely)" and "use indiscriminable contingencies" (Stokes & Baer, 1977; Stokes & Osnes, 1986) that suggest, at least implicitly, that applied generalization results from lessening control over responding. The present authors' perspective emphasizes that strong stimulus control is the primary factor in producing the precise responding required to meet the challenges of functional responding in the community.

In part, the failure to extend a stimulus control analysis to the applied problem of generalization may result from the way in which the process has been characterized in the basic research literature. Traditional descriptions of stimulus control within the basic experimental analysis of behavior literature present it as a process in opposition to stimulus generalization (Honig & Urcuioli, 1981; Terrace, 1966). The steepening of generalization gradients around an S+ that occurs following discrimination training is interpreted as increased stimulus control (Hanson, 1959, 1961; Jenkins & Harrison, 1960). Such steepening also reflects reduced stimulus generalization around the S+. However, as Stokes and Baer (1977) noted, analyses of the problem of applied generalization do not necessarily fit the traditional conceptualizations of stimulus generalization. Not only does generalization in applied situations call for active programming efforts, but also such generalization does not result simply from indiscriminate responding. For applied generalization to be functional, learners must be able to discriminate between appropriate and inappropriate performance conditions within potentially large sets of nontrained conditions that they may face in the natural community.

The key to extending stimulus control to the applied problem of generalization is a shift in focus from simple Stimulus → Response relationships to the development of control over responding by stimulus classes (Becker, Engelmann, & Thomas, 1975; Horner et al., 1982, 1984). Figure 1 presents this shift graphically, with the top panel reflecting the traditional view of stimulus control and the bottom panel representing control by a class of stimuli. Stimuli or stimulus conditions that share a critical set of characteristics (i.e., those inside the circle in the bottom panel in Figure 1) are viewed as members of a stimulus class. Stimuli or stimulus conditions that share none, or only some, of those characteristics (i.e., those outside the circle in Figure 1) are not members of that class (Becker et al., 1975).

Those critical characteristics that define a stimulus class are the "relevant" features that should control responding. When responding is brought under the control of these relevant features, *all* members of the stimulus class control responding because all members share these class-defining characteristics. Although members may differ on "irrelevant" features (i.e., characteristics that do not define membership in the stimulus class), each becomes a discriminative stimulus (S^D) that sets the occasion for the target response to occur. Because stimuli that are not members of the stimulus class do not contain all of the relevant features that define the class, they are not discriminative stimuli for the target response. Therefore, responding does not occur in the presence of stimuli or stimulus conditions that are outside the circle.

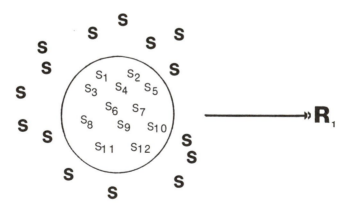

Figure 1.   Top panel: Diagram of the traditional view of a stimulus control relationship between a single discriminative stimulus and response. Bottom panel: Diagram of a stimulus control relationship between a stimulus class and response. All stimuli within the circle control responding.

Consider as an example teaching use of fast food restaurants. One could identify the relevant features that define a fast food restaurant (e.g., food ordered and picked up at a counter or window; a wait of less than 1–2 minutes for food; food delivered ready to eat), creating a stimulus class that includes any restaurant with those features. These member restaurants will differ on irrelevant features such as building color and shape, but they share the class-defining relevant features. Establishments that do not contain all relevant features (e.g., food ordered from waitress/waiter when seated; food obtained cafeteria style; food microwaved by purchaser before eating) would be outside the "fast food" stimulus class. The goal of instruction here is to establish precise responding so that the learner can successfully use any fast food restaurant, but at the same time will learn enough about the stimulus class so that he or she does not walk into a sit-down restaurant and place an order with the host/hostess at the cash register.

The "Direct Instruction" approach of Engelmann, Becker, Carnine, and their associates is a teaching technology specifically developed to bring responding under the control of stimulus classes (Becker et al., 1975; Carnine & Becker, 1982; Engelmann & Carnine, 1982). The purpose of the approach is to teach "general case" responding (i.e., responding that occurs across all members of a stimulus class after instruction on only some of those members) (Becker & Engelmann, 1978). Direct Instruction guidelines provide specific information regarding the selection and sequencing of teaching examples to produce general case responding.

General case programming (Albin et al., 1987; Horner, McDonnell, & Bellamy, 1986; Horner et al., 1982) adapts and applies Direct Instruction guidelines for teaching community skills and activities to persons with severe disabilities. Detailed procedural guidelines are presented for bringing adaptive behaviors under the control of predefined stimulus classes. Using general case programming procedures, responding across a range of nontrained conditions or settings has been shown for tasks such as street crossing (Horner, Jones, & Williams, 1985), using vending machines (Sprague & Horner, 1984), making and receiving telephone calls (Horner, Williams, & Steveley, 1987), grocery item selection (Horner, Albin, & Ralph, 1986; McDonnell & Horner, 1985), table bussing (Horner, Eberhard, & Sheehan, 1986), using soap dispensers (Pancsofar & Bates, 1985), and dressing (Day & Horner, 1986).

The general case approach offers recommendations both for ensuring that generalized responding occurs across the full range of appropriate conditions *and* that it does not occur in inappropriate conditions. Horner et al. (1982) note that general case programming involves six basic steps, as follows:

1. Define the instructional universe.
2. Define the range of relevant stimulus and response variation within that universe.

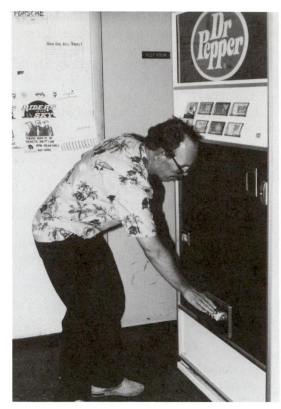

This worker's ability to perform with precision in the community adds greatly to the pleasures of an afternoon work break.

3. Select examples from the instructional universe for use in teaching and probe testing.
4. Sequence teaching examples.
5. Teach the examples.
6. Test with nontrained probe examples. (p. 74)

Specific guidelines and procedures for designing and implementing general case programs have been presented elsewhere (Albin et al., 1987; Horner, McDonnell, & Bellamy, 1986; Horner et al., 1982).

The first four of these steps in general case programming represent the crucial preparation necessary in programming for successful generalization. It is during these steps that the desired scope of generalized responding is established. The relevant stimuli defining the stimulus class that should control responding are identified, and the range of variation present in those relevant stimuli is determined. Variations in target response topographies are also determined. This analysis allows for the selection of specific teaching examples that will teach this range of variation. Guidelines for sequencing these examples are also a part of general case procedures. Success in teaching precise generalized responding depends heavily on these preparatory steps. The teaching involved in general case programming utilizes the same well-established instructional techniques (e.g., prompting, assisting, and reinforcing correct performance; ensuring good error correction; using good instructional pacing) that are used in any high-quality teaching. It is the analysis steps, those procedures that lead to the selection of optimal teaching examples and the best possible sequencing for those examples, that distinguish general case programming from other generalization strategies.

TEACHING EXAMPLES

The term *teaching examples* refers to the stimuli presented on a particular instructional opportunity or trial. Just as basic researchers utilize two types of stimuli, S+ and S−, to establish precise stimulus control (Hanson, 1959, 1961; Jenkins & Harrison, 1960), practitioners seeking to establish precise generalization in applied situations must use two types of teaching examples, positive and negative. Positive teaching examples teach the learner both how to perform a target skill or activity, and the set of conditions in which it is appropriate to perform that skill or activity. All members of the stimulus class that should control performance of the target skill or activity are potential positive teaching examples. Negative teaching examples are presented to teach the learner the conditions in which performance is not appropriate or in which some alternative response should be made. The term *negative* refers to the characteristics of the teaching examples, *not* to the instructional procedures used when teaching with them. Negative teaching examples are not members of the stimulus class that should control the target response.

Negative teaching examples are further differentiated according to their similarity with members of the class of positive examples. Similarity can be viewed as a continuous variable that depends on the number of relevant features shared by negative and positive examples. At one extreme are "maximum difference" negative examples, which are very different from and contain none of the relevant features that define positive examples. As the number of relevant features shared by negative and positive examples increases, the similarity increases. At the other extreme are "minimum difference" negative examples, which contain all but one of the relevant features that define the stimulus class of positive examples.

For example, consider potential examples that could be used in teaching a nonreader to board the proper city bus at a curbside bus stop where many buses and other vehicles stop. Taxicabs, delivery trucks, and passenger cars differ markedly from a city bus and could be used as maximum difference negative examples. A yellow school bus shares more relevant "bus" features, but also differs from the target city bus on enough relevant features to be in the middle of a similarity continuum. City buses from different routes, differentiated only by bus number and destination name, share the most relevant features with the target bus and would serve as minimum difference negative examples on the continuum. For example, correct performance may require the rider to board the "#31A—City View" bus rather than the "#31B—Bailey Hill" bus. Identical in all other relevant features, the 31B bus stands at the end of the continuum as the most similar, minimum difference negative teaching example for the 31A bus.

Using Positive and Negative Teaching Examples in General Case Programming

Horner, Eberhard, and Sheehan (1986) presented an example of using positive and negative teaching examples to teach generalized responding in an activity that required differentiating between when to and when not to bus tables in a cafeteria-type restaurant. It was equally important that students bus tables in appropriate situations *and that they not* bus tables when faced with situations where bussing was not appropriate. Training occurred on four positive examples that sampled the range of conditions in which bussing was appropriate, and on two negative examples that presented alternative conditions in which bussing was not appropriate.

Figure 2 presents Horner, Eberhard, and Sheehan's (1986) results. Following general case training, the students correctly bussed or refrained from bussing a substantial percentage (80%–100%) of 15 nontrained tables (10 to be bussed and 5 not to be bussed) in two nontrained restaurants. General case training procedures were successful in teaching students with disabilities both when and when not to perform an adaptive activity in community settings.

When Are Negative Teaching Examples Needed?

When performance settings require discriminations between conditions where responding is appropriate or inappropriate, negative teaching examples must be used during training. Negative examples provide the precision in responding demanded by such discriminations by focusing learner attention on the specific relevant features distinguishing positive examples from negative examples. However, not all skills and activities taught to learners with severe disabilities require discriminations between performance conditions. Also, strategies that are used to support the performance of learners with severe disabilities in the community may eliminate the need for discriminations. It is important that

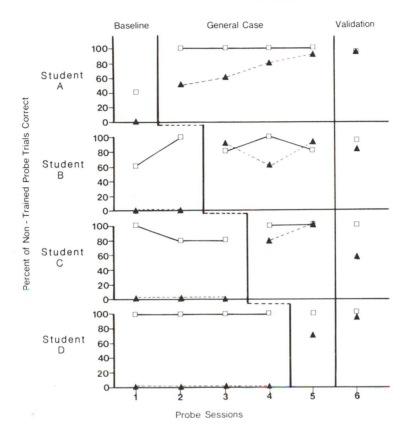

Figure 2. Percentage of nontrained "to-be-bussed" and "not-to-be-bussed" tables responded to correctly during probe sessions. (Reprinted by permission of Sage Publications, Inc., from Horner, R.H., Eberhard, J., & Sheehan, M.R. [1986]. Teaching generalized table bussng: The importance of negative teaching examples. *Behavior Modification, 10,* 457–471. Copyright © 1986 by Sage Publications, Inc.)

practitioners analyze the demands of performance settings for targeted skills and activities, and that they recognize when negative teaching examples are needed. Then, when negative examples are needed, trainers must ensure that learners receive training on a set of negative examples that is adequate to meet those demands.

The authors' experience suggests at least three general types of situations related to negative examples that practitioners may face. These situations are differentiated by two features. The first is whether correct responding requires discriminating conditions where performance is appropriate from those where it is inappropriate. If discriminations must be made, negative teaching examples are needed. The second feature distinguishes two types of situations in which negative examples are needed on the basis of how the presentation of teaching examples occurs. Each of these three situations is described in the paragraphs following.

Responding Is Always Appropriate   Regarding the first type of teaching situation, already noted, for some skills and activities, learners with disabilities experience opportunities to respond only under conditions where responding is always appropriate. Because no discriminations are required of the learner, negative teaching examples are not needed. Horner and McDonald (1982) provided an example of such a situation involving a vocational task. Students were trained to crimp/cut electronic capacitors using general case programming procedures. The instructional universe for these students included a variety of capacitors of varying size, shape, color, lead width, and lead strength. However, a critical feature of this instructional universe was that every member was to be crimp/cut. The task was one in which the learner was given only capacitors that were to be treated similarly (i.e., crimp/cut to the same specifications). Because the learner never needed to discriminate between conditions where responding was appropriate versus inappropriate, only a range of positive examples was needed to teach the desired general case responding.

Performance aspects of many tasks (e.g., the need for specialized materials or equipment, limits on the scope of the instructional universe targeted, the existence of external support mechanisms to screen performance opportunities) may eliminate the need for negative teaching examples. However, it is unlikely (and certainly undesirable) that all instructional objectives will target skills or activities that fit this situation. Attempts to simplify or control the complexities of the natural environment may limit the impact that newly learned skills and activities have on the life-styles of persons with severe disabilities. Practitioners cannot overlook the need for using negative examples in instruction designed to teach the discriminations demanded by the natural environment.

Training Setting Naturally Presents Negative Examples   In terms of the second type of teaching situation, for some tasks that require discriminations between appropriate and inappropriate response conditions, the training setting(s) naturally presents a range of conditions in which differential responding must occur. As a result, the trainer's job is made a bit easier. The training setting ensures that learners will experience at least some negative teaching examples because they occur naturally. The main concern in this type of situation is to ensure that the training setting provides a sufficient number and range of negative examples to adequately teach the desired skill or activity.

The skill of street crossing fits this type of situation when training occurs in the community (Horner et al., 1985). The leaner must be able to discriminate conditions when it is appropriate to cross from those when it is inappropriate. Training on streets in the community results in a naturally occurring variety of examples of both types of conditions. Although the natural variety presented by the community may be adequate, it is possible that the community may fail to present at least some conditions or may present conditions at too low a frequency to teach fully the desired scope for this skill. Trainers must monitor the teaching examples experienced, to ensure an adequate range of both positive and negative examples. For example, a trainer might need to arrange to have cars pulling away from the curb, cars exiting a nearby parking lot, or motorcycles circling the block, so that sufficient numbers of training trials occur with these conditions.

Practitioner Specifically Programs All Teaching Examples The third type of situation faced in training skills or activities to learners with disabilities is one in which the program designer/trainer specifically programs all teaching examples. Rather than allowing the environment to naturally present teaching trials, the practitioner controls the presentation of both positive and negative teaching examples. In this type of situation, it is easy to overlook the need for negative examples. There is a tendency to focus on instruction with positive teaching examples, prompting and/or assisting correct performance in appropriate conditions and providing reinforcement for it. Because the trainer controls the presentation of teaching examples, he or she often uses this control to avoid or eliminate conditions in which responding is not appropriate. However, when training concludes, this artificial control is no longer present, and the learner suddenly may be faced with conditions in which the target response is not appropriate. Unfortunately, the learner has not received instruction on these negative examples, and errors result.

Finding and selecting grocery items using some type of picture cue list illustrates this third situation. Often a set of target ("positive") items is designated, and training begins to teach a learner to find and select those items. The trainer assists and prompts early in instruction to minimize errors, such as the selection of incorrect items. The trainee learns to find and select positive items, but he or she receives no experience discriminating those items from other items that share similar features ("negative" items). If negative teaching examples are presented at all, they are the result of learner errors (e.g., selecting incorrect items), rather than systematic analysis by the trainer. When this learner shops independently following training, conditions may be such that he or she selects a similar-looking negative item rather than a particular target item.

Several of the generalization errors observed in grocery item selection by McDonnell and Horner (1985) fit this pattern. Students in this study received positive trials in selecting 15 grocery items based on picture cues. They also were trained to make an overt verbal or nonverbal "not there" response when a target item was out of stock (i.e., its spot on the shelf was empty). However, no planned negative teaching examples related to discriminating among items were presented during training. Although students were able to find a substantial percentage of the target items in the nontrained generalization probe stores, one of the frequent error patterns observed was the selection of incorrect items that shared some relevant features with the target item (e.g., same brand but different product; same product but different brand) when that target item was not in stock or was not readily located.

GUIDELINES FOR SELECTING AND SEQUENCING NEGATIVE TEACHING EXAMPLES

Three basic guidelines are offered here for selecting negative teaching examples when they are needed to teach generalization with precision:

1. Select maximum difference negative teaching examples in order to quickly teach that differential responding is needed.
2. Select minimum difference negative teaching examples in order to teach the precise discriminations that are necessary for correct responding.
3. Select minimum difference negative teaching examples that minimize generalization errors due to restricted stimulus control.

To date, research involving persons with severe handicaps suggests that both maximum and minimum difference negative teaching examples should be included when negative teaching examples are needed in instruction. A logical analysis of instruction supports this conclusion as well. The two types of negative examples serve different purposes in instructional sequences. Maximum difference negative examples provide easy opportunities to teach learners that differential responding is required in a skill or activity. Minimum difference negative examples provide opportunities to teach learners the precise discriminations that must be made for successful performance of that skill or activity. Each of the three guidelines is discussed in the subsections following.

Select Maximum Difference Negative Teaching Examples

Although there are no conclusive data indicating that maximum difference negative examples are necessary to teach precise generalized responding, both the authors' experience and a logical analysis of the problem faced by learners with severe disabilities support this guideline. The primary rationale for this guideline is based on the logistics of teaching learners with severe disabilities that discriminations and differential responses are needed for correct performance of many community skills and activities. For example, in several research studies utilizing tasks that required differential responding, the authors have observed that many participants show pretraining response patterns characterized by a single, predominant response tendency (Albin, 1986/1987; Horner, Albin, & Ralph, 1986; Horner, Eberhard, & Sheehan, 1986). For correct performance, this initial tendency for a single response must be replaced by a pattern of differential responding that is based on discriminating between appropriate and inappropraite response conditions. Maximum difference negative examples are more readily discriminated from positive examples, and, as a result, they increase the speed with which differential responding develops.

A second reason for including maximum difference negative examples is that they are useful in teaching learners the range of conditions in which responding is inappropriate. Just as positive teaching examples are selected to sample the range of conditions in which responding should occur (Horner et al., 1982), negative teaching examples must teach the range of conditions where responding is inappropriate. Both maximum and minimum difference negative examples may be needed to adequately represent this range to learners with severe disabilities.

Select Minimum Difference Negative Teaching Examples

In designing and implementing instruction for persons with severe disabilities, a likely problem is the failure to include adequate minimum difference negative examples. Often only maximum difference negative examples are utilized in an attempt to promote skill acquisition and to minimize learner errors. Discriminations are easier to learn, and acquisition may occur rapidly. Under some conditions generalized responding may also occur. However, the learner may not be able to perform with the precision needed to meet the demands of natural performance conditions.

Horner, Albin, and Ralph (1986) demonstrated the need for minimum difference negative teaching examples in teaching precise grocery selection skills. Two sets of teaching examples were used to teach learners with disabilities to select 10 grocery items from pictures that served as a shopping list. Both sets contained the same 10 target items (i.e., positive teaching examples). The difference between the two sets was the negative teaching examples used in each. One set used negative examples for each target item that shared relevant stimulus features with that item (i.e., minimum difference negative examples). The other set utilized as negative examples only items that shared no relevant features with a particular target item (i.e., maximum difference negative examples.)

Testing in Horner, Albin, and Ralph (1986) involved 30 grocery item trials, one with each of the 10 positive target items and 20 trials with nontrained

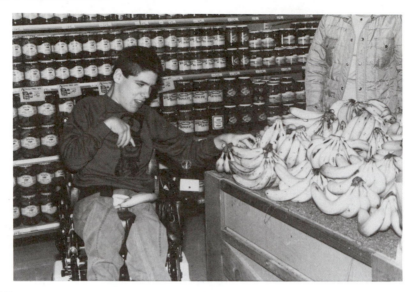

Although grocery stores present many difficult discriminations, the unique features of some grocery items make them readily recognizable.

incorrect items that were minimally different from the target items (two minimum difference negatives for each target item). These generalization test probes occurred in a nontrained grocery store. Participants were given a positive item picture and their attention was directed to a particular item, either a target item or one of the two minimum difference negative items for that pictured item.

Figure 3 presents the generalization test probe results from Horner, Albin, and Ralph (1986). Participants successfully selected the 10 positive items regardless of the set of examples used in training. However, only when participants were trained with minimum difference negative teaching examples were they able to correctly reject a substantial number of the nontrained minimum difference test probe items. Participants trained only with maximum difference negative examples looked at a picture of a positive item and then consistently selected an incorrect item that shared several features with, but was not, the pictured item. Training with minimum difference negative examples was necessary to produce the precision in responding required for correct performance in the nontrained grocery store.

Select Minimum Difference Negative Teaching Examples that Minimize Restricted Stimulus Control

Generalization failures, the errors that occur in nontrained conditions after acquisition criteria have been met, provide practitioners with valuable informa-

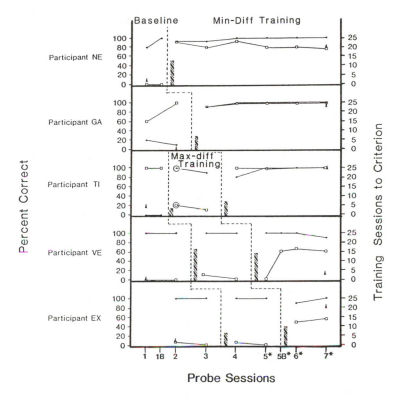

Figure 3.   Percentage of correct selections and rejections of grocery store probe items. (Reprinted with permission, from Horner, R.H., Albin, R.W., & Ralph, G. [1986]. Generalization with precision: The role of negative teaching examples in the instruction of generalized grocery item selection. *Journal of The Association for Persons with Severe Handicaps, 11,* 300–308. Copyright 1986 by The Association for Persons with Severe Handicaps.)

tion (Horner et al., 1984). Rather than simply being random, such errors frequently reflect a consistent pattern of incorrect generalized responding. Such patterns focus attention on the inadequacies of training that produced the underlying stimulus control problem(s). Understanding why error patterns occur provides valuable information for designing instruction that avoids generalization errors, or remediates them if they already exist (Engelmann & Carnine, 1982; Horner et al., 1984).

Horner et al. (1984) identified four error patterns drawn from their analysis of the applied generalization literature. They described these patterns as follows: 1) irrelevant stimuli control the target response, 2) irrelevant stimuli control irrelevant competing responses, 3) limited variations of the target response, and 4) restricted stimulus control. The restricted stimulus control error pattern especially merits elaboration here, as it presents a direct challenge to a technology of instruction involving negative teaching examples. It is the one pattern that results directly from inadequate use of minimum difference negative teaching examples.

Restricted Stimulus Control Restricted stimulus control errors occur in situations in which reponding should be under the control of conjunctive features of a compound stimulus. For example, in shelving grocery items, brand label, product, and package size are all relevant for correct performance. Similarly, color and fabric type are relevant to the correct sorting of clothing at a commercial laundry. If training results in responding that is controlled by only one feature or a subset of features of the relevant compound, generalization errors will occur.

At the heart of restricted stimulus control errors are conditions in which stimuli containing some, but not all, of the elements of a relevant stimulus compound are present. These conditions should be treated as negative examples (i.e., no target response or a differential response is made). When restricted control exists, they are treated as positive examples (i.e., the target response is made), and an error results. Avoiding this problem requires training that includes minimum difference negative teaching examples that contain some, but not all, of the relevant compound elements. By setting up conditional discriminations involving these negative examples, the precision of instruction matches the precision demands in performance settings.

Albin (1986/1987) demonstrated the role of negative teaching examples in remediating restricted stimulus control errors in learners with moderate and severe mental retardation. Two companion studies were conducted using generalized performance of vocational tasks as the dependent variable. In each study, two sets of teaching examples were used to train the vocational tasks, inserting electronic resistors into circuit boards in Study 1 and reshelving grocery items in Study 2. In each task, correct responding required control by a two-element conjunctive stimulus compound: size and color of the resistors, and brand label and a second feature that varied across grocery items (e.g., label and product picture, label and product color, label and container shape, label and container size).

Each set of teaching examples shared a common set of positive examples. The difference between the two sets was the way negative teaching examples were selected. In one set, negative examples shared irrelevant features with positive examples, but they contained neither of the two relevant stimulus features. These were termed *zero-feature* negative examples. In the second set, negative examples contained one or the other, but not both, features that made up the relevant stimulus compound. These were termed *one-feature* negative examples. Based on the logic of a stimulus control analysis, instruction that involved only zero-feature negative examples is likely to result in generalization errors due to restricted stimulus control. Negative examples that contain the controlling subset of relevant features would be treated as positive examples.

Results from both studies showed that generalization errors made by participants trained only with zero-feature negative examples were likely to reflect problems due to restricted stimulus control. This was best illustrated in the study that used the resistor insertion task. This task involved correctly determining where to insert a resistor based on the relevant stimulus features of size (small) and color (brown). Small, brown resistors were to be inserted into one circuit board, and all other resistors into another. Data were collected periodically with a set of nontrained probe resistors that included four types: 1) small and brown, 2) neither small nor brown, 3) small but not brown, and 4) brown but not small. Figure 4 shows the nontrained probe resistors.

Four participants with severe disabilities were trained to insert the resistors. Initially, training included only small, brown resistors (positive examples) and resistors that were neither small nor brown (zero-feature negative examples). It was anticipated that the participants would learn that either size or color was important, rather than that a combination of size and color was important.

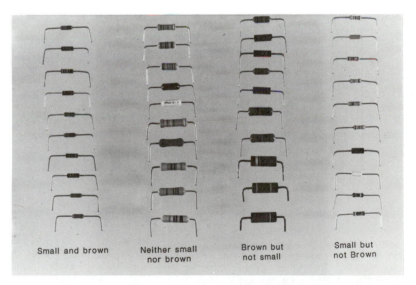

Small and brown   Neither small nor brown   Brown but not small   Small but not Brown

Figure 4. Set of nontrained probe resistors used by Albin (1986/1987) to assess restricted stimulus control.

This would result in participants not doing well when presented with the precision demands of the full set of probe resistors. As can be seen in Figure 5, this prediction proved accurate. After training with zero-feature negatives, participants showed significant improvement over pretraining baseline performance on three types of probe resistors. However, on the small but not brown probe resistors, the four participants continued to have problems, making substantially more errors than on any of the other three types. This pattern suggests that size alone was controlling responding and that all small resistors, regardless of color, were treated similarly. This restricted stimulus control resulted in correct performance on resistors that were small and brown, neither small nor brown, and brown but not small, but it produced incorrect overgeneralization to small but not brown resistors (i.e., one-feature small negative examples).

After the initial training that included only zero-feature negative examples, participants received additional training using small but not brown, and brown but not small, resistors as negative teaching examples (i.e., both possible types of one-feature negative examples). When tested again with the nontrained probe resistors, the frequency of generalization errors on the one-feature small probe resistors was reduced. The results in Figure 5 indicate only small differences in errors on the four types of resistors after participants were

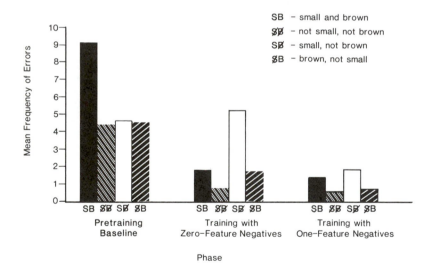

Figure 5. Mean frequency of errors on each type of nontrained probe resistor during Pretraining Baseline, Training with Zero-Feature Negatives, and Training with One-Feature Negative phases. Means are from four participants in the first two phases and from three participants in the third phase. One participant was dropped from the Training with One-Feature Negatives phase because of behavior problems. (Adapted from Albin [1986/1987].)

trained with the one-feature negative examples that avoided the restricted stimulus control problem.

Findings consistent with those reported by Albin (1986/1987) have been observed by other researchers working on the problem of restricted stimulus control and the related phenomenon of stimulus overselectivity in persons with autism (see Schreibman, Chapter 2, in this book). Conditional discrimination training similar to that used by Albin (1986/1987) reduced stimulus overselectivity in children with autism (Schreibman, Charlop, & Koegel, 1982) and in children and adolescents with mental retardation (Allen & Fuqua, 1985). Both of those studies used a discrimination task involving compound visual stimuli. When S − 's contained none of the relevant features of the compound S + , learner responding was controlled by only a single feature of the relevant stimulus compound. When S − 's contained some, but not all, of the relevant features, restricted stimulus control (i.e., overselectivity) was eliminated.

RESEARCH IMPLICATIONS OF
NEGATIVE TEACHING EXAMPLES

The broad definition and such strategies as "train loosely" and "use indiscriminable contingencies" presented by Stokes and Baer (1977) are often interpreted as suggesting that generalization occurs through a loosening of control over responding. In fact, to meet the performance demands of natural environments, the opposite is true. Functional generalization in applied settings requires very precise control over responding. Emphasis on stimulus control highlights this need for precision in applied generalization settings. Application of stimulus control principles to the problem of generalization in applied settings has important implications both for how researchers and practitioners assess generalization and for the dependent variables used in generalization research.

Assess Generalization across Full Range of Conditions

To solve the applied problem of generalization, responding must occur across the full range of appropriate conditions, and not occur across all inappropriate conditions (Horner et al., 1984). Determining the success of generalization efforts requires assessment that adequately samples this range of conditions. The real world is a demanding performance environment that frequently requires the ability to discriminate whether and/or how to respond. Too often practitioners and researchers lose sight of the fact that functional generalization is not simply indiscriminate generalization. One major result of this is the tendency to assess generalized responding only under a very limited set of conditions in which responding is appropriate (Kayser & Billingsley, 1986).

Generalization failures related to problems with negative teaching examples are observed only when performance is tested under "negative" performance conditions. Learners may show excellent generalization in nontrained conditions in which responding should occur, but they may be equally likely to respond in conditions in which such responding is inappropriate. Only by assessing generalization across a full range of conditions, both "positive" and "negative," can the precision of responding be accurately judged.

Use Whole Task Success/Failure as the Dependent Variable

A focus on the precision of generalized responding also has implications for the dependent variable used in research on generalization. Often practitioners and researchers emphasize percentage of task analysis steps completed correctly in measuring for generalization. Research on the role of negative examples in general case programming indicates the importance of percentage of correct performance across a range of nontrained conditions as a dependent variable that directly assesses generalization in applied settings. Learners trained only with maximum difference negative examples in Horner, Albin, and Ralph (1986) or only with zero-feature negative examples in Albin (1986/1987) performed all but one task step correctly in situations in which overgeneralization errors occurred. Unfortunately, that one step was a failure to make the critical discrimination on whether to respond. Attention only to percentage of task analysis steps performed correctly may result in the false perception that generalized responding is "good" (i.e., a high percentage of steps is completed), when, in fact, failure on a critical step means that performance cannot meet the demands of the natural environment (cf. Aeschlemann & Schladenhauffen, 1984).

SUMMARY

Practitioners face a major challenge when they endeavor to teach generalized skills and activities to persons with severe disabilities. Success in community settings requires generalization with precision across a range of nontrained appropriate and inappropriate performance conditions. General case programming offers a technology of generalization, based on stimulus control principles, that meets these precision demands. A critical feature of this technology is the optimal use of teaching examples, including negative teaching examples, to teach the discriminations between performance conditions so often required in community settings. In teaching community tasks, practitioners should identify when such discriminations are needed, and select negative examples that teach the learner to attend and respond only to the relevant stimuli that define the discrimination. Teaching generalized behaviors has life-style impact only when those behaviors generalize with the precision required by natural settings.

REFERENCES

Aeschlemann, S.R., & Schladenhauffen, J. (1984). Acquisition, generalization, and maintenance of grocery shopping skills by severely mentally retarded adolescents. *Mental Retardation, 5*, 245–258.

Albin, R.W. (1987). The role of negative teaching examples in the development of conjunctive stimulus control with learners experiencing moderate and severe mental retardation (Doctoral dissertation, University of Oregon, Eugene, 1986). *Dissertation Abstracts International, 47*, 3392-A.

Albin, R.W., McDonnell, J.J., & Wilcox, B. (1987). Designing interventions to meet activity goals. In B. Wilcox & G.T. Bellamy, *A comprehensive guide to* The Activities Catalog: *An alternative curriculum for youth and adults with severe disabilities* (pp. 63–88). Baltimore: Paul H. Brookes Publishing Co.

Allen, K.D., & Fuqua, R.W. (1985). Eliminating selective stimulus control: A comparison of two procedures for teaching mentally retarded children to respond to compound stimuli. *Journal of Experimental Child Psychology, 39*, 55–71.

Becker, W.C., & Engelmann, S.E. (1978). Systems for basic instruction: Theory and applications. In A. Catania & T. Brigham (Eds.), *Handbook of applied behavior analysis: Social and instructional processes* (pp. 325–378). New York: Irvington.

Becker, W.C., Engelmann, S., & Thomas, D. (1975). *Teaching 2: Cognitive learning and instruction.* Chicago: Science Research Associates.

Bellamy, G.T., Horner, R.H., & Inman, D. (1979). *Vocational habilitation of severely retarded adults: A direct service technology.* Baltimore: University Park Press.

Carnine, D.W., & Becker, W.C. (1982). Theory of instruction: Generalisation issues. *Educational Psychology, 2*, 249–262.

Day, H.M., & Horner, R.H. (1986). Response variation and the generalization of dressing skills. *Applied Research in Mental Retardation, 7*, 189–202.

Engelmann, S., & Carnine, D.W. (1982). *Theory of instruction: Principles and applications.* New York: Irvington.

Hanson, H.M. (1959). Effects of discrimination training on stimulus generalization. *Journal of Experimental Psychology, 58*, 321–334.

Hanson, H.M. (1961). Stimulus generalization following three-stimulus discrimination training. *Journal of Comparative and Physiological Psychology, 54*, 181–185.

Honig, W.K., & Urcuioli, P.J. (1981). The legacy of Guttman and Kalish (1956): 25 years of research on stimulus generalization. *Journal of the Experimental Analysis of Behavior, 36*, 405–445.

Horner, R.H., Albin, R.W., & Ralph, G. (1986). Generalization with precision: The role of negative teaching examples in the instruction of generalized grocery item selection. *Journal of The Association for Persons with Severe Handicaps, 11*, 300–308.

Horner, R.H., Bellamy, G.T., & Colvin, G.T. (1984). Responding in the presence of nontrained stimuli: Implications of generalization error patterns. *Journal of The Association for Persons with Severe Handicaps, 9*, 287–296.

Horner, R.H., Eberhard, J., & Sheehan, M.R. (1986). Teaching generalized table bussing: The importance of negative teaching examples. *Behavior Modification, 10*, 457–471.

Horner, R.H., Jones, D., & Williams, J.A. (1985). A functional approach to teaching generalized street crossing. *Journal of The Association for Persons with Severe Handicaps, 10*, 71–78.

Horner, R.H., & McDonald, R.S. (1982). A comparison of single instance and general case instruction in teaching a generalized vocational skill. *Journal of The Association for the Severely Handicapped, 7,* 7–20.

Horner, R.H., McDonnell, J.J., & Bellamy, G.T. (1986). Teaching generalized skills: General case instruction in simulation and community settings. In R.H. Horner, L.H. Meyer, & H.D. Fredericks (Eds.), *Education of learners with severe handicaps: Exemplary service strategies* (pp. 289–314). Baltimore: Paul H. Brookes Publishing Co.

Horner, R.H., Sprague, J., & Wilcox, B. (1982). Constructing general case programs for community activities. In B. Wilcox & G.T. Bellamy (Eds.), *Design of high school programs for severely handicapped students* (pp. 61–98). Baltimore: Paul H. Brookes Publishing Co.

Horner, R.H., Williams, J.A., & Steveley, J.D. (1987). Acquisition of generalized telephone use by students with moderate and severe mental retardation. *Research in Developmental Disabilities, 8,* 229–247.

Jenkins, H.M., & Harrison, R.H. (1960). Effect of discrimination training on auditory generalization. *Journal of Experimental Psychology, 59,* 246–253.

Kayser, J.E., & Billingsley, F.F. (1986). Generalization: A review of assessment procedures. In N. Haring (Principal Investigator), *Investigating the problem of skill generalization: Literature review III* (U.S. Department of Education, Contract No. 300-82-0364) (pp. 1–38). Seattle: University of Washington, College of Education.

Marholin, D., II, & Touchette, P.E. (1979). The role of stimulus control and response consequences. In A. Goldstein & F. Kanfer (Eds.), *Maximizing treatment gains* (pp. 303–351). New York: Academic Press.

McDonnell, J.J., & Horner, R.H. (1985). Effects of in vivo and simulation-plus-in vivo training on the acquisition and generalization of a grocery item search strategy by high school students with severe handicaps. *Analysis and Intervention in Developmental Disabilities, 5,* 323–343.

Pancsofar, E.L., & Bates, P. (1985). The impact of the acquisition of successive training exemplars on generalization. *Journal of The Association for Persons with Severe Handicaps, 10,* 95–104.

Schreibman, L., Charlop, M.H., & Koegel, R.L. (1982). Teaching autistic children to use extra-stimulus prompts. *Journal of Experimental Child Psychology, 33,* 475–491.

Sprague, J.R., & Horner, R.H. (1984). The effects of single instance, multiple instance, and general case training on generalized vending machine use by moderately and severely handicapped students. *Journal of Applied Behavior Analysis, 17,* 273–278.

Stokes, T.F., & Baer, D.M. (1977). An implicit technology of generalization. *Journal of Applied Behavior Analysis, 10,* 349–367.

Stokes, T.F., & Osnes, P.G. (1986). Programming the generalization of children's social behavior. In P.S. Strain, M.J. Guralnick, & H. Walker (Eds.), *Children's social behavior: Development, assessment, and modification* (pp. 407–440). New York: Academic Press.

Terrace, H. (1966). Stimulus control. In W. Honig (Ed.), *Operant behavior: Areas of research and application* (pp. 271–344). New York: Appleton-Century-Crofts.

Wilcox, B., & Bellamy, G.T. (1987). *A comprehensive guide to* The Activities Catalog: *An alternative curriculum for youth and adults with severe disabilities.* Baltimore: Paul H. Brookes Publishing Co.

Chapter 6

Generalization and Maintenance of Unsupervised Responding via Remote Contingencies

Glen Dunlap and Anthony J. Plienis

While many individuals with severe developmental disabilities have learned to respond in the immediate presence of skillful supervision and clear contingencies of reinforcement, many of these same persons do not respond appropriately when they are asked to perform in unsupervised contexts. Indeed, when children (and adults) with autism or severe mental retardation are left to respond independently, they frequently revert to high frequencies of stereotypic or other nonproductive, occasionally bizarre, response patterns. This failure to generalize from training to unsupervised contexts has seriously impaired efforts to promote integration and has limited the social, residential, and educational options available to this population of severely handicapped individuals.

This chapter examines one broadly defined approach to promoting adaptive behavior in unsupervised settings. Specifically, the authors argue that a significant deficiency in the development (and education) of many developmen-

The preparation of this chapter, and portions of the research described herein, were supported by the U.S. Department of Education (Special Education Program) Contract No. 300-82-0362. However, opinions expressed by the authors do not necessarily reflect the position or policy of the U.S. Department of Education and no official endorsement should be inferred.

tally disabled learners is that they have not learned to respond on the basis of remote contingencies. While normally developing children soon learn to behave appropriately in the absence of continuous supervision or clearly visible rewards, children with severe handicaps often behave appropriately only in the presence of specifically structured and highly predictable behavioral consequences (Dunlap & Johnson, 1985). They do not respond well when contingencies are infrequent, indistinct, or significantly delayed. However, evidence is emerging that suggests that developmentally disabled individuals can learn to respond on the basis of more remote (and more normalized) contingencies. This chapter reviews that evidence, discusses the implications for community integration, and suggests some directions of study that might benefit from further applied research.

OVERVIEW OF UNSUPERVISED PERFORMANCE

Independent, unsupervised performance is an important attribute for members of all populations, regardless of handicap. Most people, unburdened by significant disabilities, are able to perform previously learned skills independently. Although the rate and quality of performance may vary in accordance with a number of motivational and setting factors, nonhandicapped children and adults will usually respond in an adaptive manner so long as there is a sufficiently compelling reason (i.e., contingency) to do so.

Even the most casual inspection of a normal child's functioning produces numerous examples of behavior that are influenced by delayed contingencies. For example, household chores are performed independently because a weekly allowance is contingent upon task completion (or, perhaps, to avoid a parent's criticism). The reward (or punisher) is not likely to be issued immediately, but the child has learned to anticipate its eventual delivery.

As normal children develop, their behavior comes under the influence of increasingly remote contingencies. Very young children require frequent rewards and reminders of behavioral guidelines. By the teenage years, most well-practiced behavior is maintained by very lean schedules of reinforcement and by subtle, often extremely remote, consequences. Adults, of course, complete daily routines and work long hours for rewards that are often difficult to identify and that are usually very distant. Our society is structured to expect a great deal of adaptive, conforming behavior for meager allotments of explicit reinforcers. In other words, a prerequisite of most social participation is the ability to behave acceptably without continuous reinforcement and supervision.

Persons with severe developmental disabilities face significant obstacles in their efforts to participate in the mainstream of the community. Their communication skills are extremely restricted and/or disordered, and their related patterns of interpersonal responses are often similarly inappropriate. Most lack a standard repertoire of self-care skills, and few have developed socially accepted leisure or recreational skills. In addition, many individuals with autism and/or severe mental retardation display excess behaviors (such as stereotypies, aggression, and tantrums), which can impede the process of skill development (Koegel & Covert, 1972) and seriously disrupt community participation. Fortunately, years of research and practice have provided means to teach functional skills and to reduce or eliminate many excess behaviors (Horner, Meyer, & Fredericks, 1986; Koegel, Rincover, & Egel, 1982). These positive results have been produced, in virtually all instances, through careful manipulations of antecedents and consequences in the immediate environment (Lovaas & Newsom, 1976). Research has shown that so long as such stimuli are arranged in specific ways, these favorable behaviors can be maintained. In other words, so long as educators or other training personnel can provide for an effectively supportive environment, desirable performances can be anticipated.

A missing step in this process involves the assurance that functional, socially acceptable behavior will be exhibited and maintained when specialized trainers are not available to guarantee environmental support. Without such assurance, persons with severe handicaps will continue to fail at an alarming rate when they encounter normalized community expectations. Consider, for example, a young man with autism who has learned a complex assembly task in his specialized high school program. He can complete the task skillfully and his performance is acceptable when his teachers are in the immediate vicinity and are providing explicit praise and redirection on a regular basis. Unfortunately, when his teachers leave the room, he gazes at the fluorescent lights, flaps his hands, and makes no progress on his work. This young man will not succeed in a workplace that is not equipped to provide continuous supervision and frequent reinforcement.

Consider also a girl whose long history of aggression was reversed by her one-to-one trainer. Using a stimulus shaping procedure and a systematically faded DRO, the trainer had eliminated aggression in his presence. However, the girl continued to display aggressive acts when the trainer was absent. As a result, she was not allowed to participate with the other children during community outings, and most of her teachers were reluctant to provide meaningful direct instruction.

The problems just described reflect a number of critical concerns for those interested in promoting the community integration of persons with severe developmental disabilities. They also exemplify the limited influence that is typically established by highly structured, behavioral programs. This limitation has been recognized for many years and has been the focus of considerable applied research activity (Stokes & Baer, 1977).

Efforts to extend the influence of training conditions to nontraining contexts have been undertaken using a variety of applied tactics (Drabman, Hammer, & Rosenbaum, 1979; Egel, 1982; Marholin & Siegel, 1978; Stokes & Baer, 1977). One general approach has been to provide training in multiple contexts with the expectation that, eventually, the effects of training would generalize to future untrained situations. This tactic has broad appeal, is well documented, and has been cited as a rationale for parent and staff training (i.e., if enough people provide functional contingencies in enough situations, generalization to other situations is likely to occur). Unfortunately, this approach also has limitations. Many persons with developmental disabilities continue to exhibit discriminated responding in training versus nontraining conditions (Koegel, Schreibman, Johnson, O'Neill, & Dunlap, 1984). In other words, even if the parents, teachers, and camp counselors are trained to use effective reinforcers in a variety of settings, this does not necessarily imply that behavior will be appropriate with the untrained job supervisor, substitute teacher, or store clerk.

Another broadly defined approach has involved the use of indiscriminable contingencies (Stokes & Baer, 1977; Stokes & Osnes, 1986). The logic underlying this approach is that the delivery of clear and immediate consequences serves to distinguish a training from a nontraining context. Thus, if contingencies can be set up so that they are both functional and difficult to detect, one could expect to see greater generalization. The use of this tactic with severely handicapped persons has been most commonly seen in the use of intermittent reinforcement schedules (e.g., Koegel & Rincover, 1977); however the use of delayed reinforcement contingencies (e.g., Fowler & Baer, 1981) also holds promise. The development and application of indiscriminable and delayed reinforcement strategies is the topic of this chapter and is discussed in detail in later sections.

APPLIED RESEARCH ON UNSUPERVISED
RESPONDING AND REMOTE CONTINGENCIES

Applied research that has directly addressed independent, unsupervised responding by persons with severe developmental disabilities is sparse. As a result, there are few clearly documented procedures for teaching severely handicapped learners to respond adaptively in unsupervised contexts. This section reviews some of the procedures and variables that have been studied.

As indicated by the introductory paragraphs of this chapter, this review is limited to applied studies of unsupervised responding (or behavior exhibited in the absence of training personnel). Thus, the chapter does not cover much of the extensive and highly relevant work on chaining, prompt fading, and intermittent reinforcement, except as these topics form the basis of and apply specifically to unsupervised behavior. The discussion is also restricted to manipulations involving remote contingencies with severely developmentally disabled individuals. Because the promising work on self-management does not yet meet these criteria, readers interested in this growing literature are referred to, for example, Browder and Shapiro (1985), Fowler, Baer, and Stolz (1984), and Liberty (1984), in addition to Chapter 3, by Koegel and Koegel, in this volume.

Discriminability, Predictability, and Unsupervised Responding

One of the most commonly recognized phenomena in behavioral training and education is the situational dependency of behavior change. As contingencies of reinforcement and punishment exert their influence over behavior, the stimuli associated with those contingencies acquire discriminative properties (Horner, Bellamy, & Colvin, 1984). The presentation of such stimuli then result in the behavioral increases (or decreases) that were produced by the contingencies. This stimulus control is often acquired by teachers, parents, and other training personnel who use effective rewards and punishers to modify behavior. Thus, behavior is apt to be different when a trainer is present versus when he or she is absent.

The stimulus control established in the process of training individuals with severe handicaps is likely to be especially striking. As discussed previously, this may be partially due to problematic learning patterns that tend to restrict the number of controlling stimuli (e.g., Dunlap, Koegel, & Burke, 1981; Lovaas, Koegel, & Schreibman, 1979). In addition, effective training usually involves highly salient and artificial stimulus characteristics that are very readily discriminated from nontraining contexts. Training activities for this population (e.g., Lovaas, 1977) often include carefully presented instructions, and, in particular, frequent and powerful consequences, such as tokens, food, sensory stimuli, or dramatic praise. As such salient reinforcers (or punishers) are almost never available in the absence of training personnel, the presence and absence of training contingencies are easily detected. Because of this clear discriminability, behavior displayed when trainers are present is often much more appropriate than when trainers are absent.

In efforts to promote generalization, many authors (Stokes & Baer, 1977; Stokes & Osnes, 1986) have advocated using indiscriminable contingencies. Such an approach typically involves intermittent or delayed schedules of reinforcement; however, discriminability may also be reduced by delivering contingencies in an unpredictable manner, meaning that no clear stimuli are present to signal the presence of contingencies.

Unpredictable (or unsignaled) contingencies may be especially useful with independent, unsupervised responding. For example, when a classroom teacher leaves the room, normally developing children may leave their assignments and "goof off" if they have a look-out or if their teachers' return will be predictably preceded by a warning signal, such as the sound of shoes on a resonant hallway floor. In contrast, if the teacher's return cannot be predicted and if contingencies are geared to the children's unsupervised responding, the children's independent behavior is apt to be much more productive (Marholin & Steinman, 1977). This observation has parallels in the animal literature (e.g., Sidman, 1953) and has been referred to by educators (e.g., Paine, Radicchi, Rosellini, Deutchman, & Darch, 1983); however, few studies have directly explored this phenomenon with handicapped populations.

In one early investigation, Risley (1968) used an unsignaled contingency to suppress the unsupervised climbing behavior of a 6-year-old girl. This girl had a lengthy history of several deviant behaviors, including aggression and climbing on bookshelves and other objects. After several procedures had failed to affect these dangerous responses, contingent punishment was applied by the trainer. The punisher rapidly eliminated climbing when the trainer was present. However, the dangerous climbing continued during 5-minute presession periods when the girl was alone. At this stage in the experiment, the trainer's presence had become a discriminative stimulus, indicating that a punisher would be applied contingent upon climbing. Similarly, the trainer's absence signaled a lack of contingencies. Observing through a one-way window, the trainer then extended the punishment contingency to these unsupervised periods. Henceforth, whenever climbing occurred, the trainer entered the room, delivered the consequence, and departed. The girl's dangerous climbing was rapidly and dramatically reduced. In subsequent reports, other researchers have employed similar manipulations of unsignaled contingencies to extend control to unsupervised contexts (e.g., Van Houten, 1986).

Dunlap and Johnson (1985) pursued the logic of unpredictable contingencies in an investigation of independent task responding by autistic children. Within multiple baseline and reversal designs, they compared the effects of two supervision strategies on the children's productivity when the children were left to work independently on assigned tasks. In the first condition, labeled "predictable supervision (PS)," the trainer was present for a period of time and then left the room without returning until the session ended. In an "unpredictable supervision" (US) condition, the trainer's presence was scheduled on a random and intermittent basis throughout the session. The total amount of time the trainer was present and providing contingent reinforcement was held constant across the two conditions. Data were collected on on-task behavior and on work completed when the trainer was present and, more importantly, when the trainer was absent.

Dunlap and Johnson's (1985) results can be summarized as follows: 1) rates of on-task productive responding when the trainer was present were consistently high under both supervision conditions (PS and US); 2) when the trainer was absent from the room in the PS condition, on-task behavior and productivity were very low across all children; however, 3) when the trainer's presence and reinforcement were scheduled to occur in an *unpredictable* manner, independent responding was always relatively high. Figure 1 summarizes some of these results. Depicted are the average rates of task completion under the PS and US conditions when the trainer was absent from the room. While each child worked on a different, individually assigned task, the results consistently illustrate the superiority of unpredictable supervision. That is, when the trainer's presence (and the availability of reinforcement) was not signaled by predictable cues or time intervals, responding in the absence of immediate supervision was markedly facilitated.

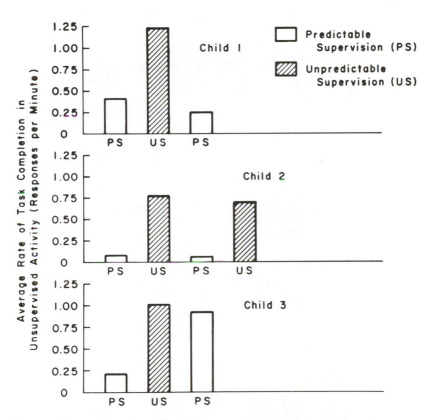

Figure 1. Rates of task completion in independent, unsupervised activity by three autistic children. Results show averaged rates under predictable and unpredictable supervision conditions (see text). Data are based on findings in Dunlap and Johnson (1985).

The results of Dunlap and Johnson's (1985) analysis and those of other researchers (e.g., Corte, Wolf, & Locke, 1971; Marholin & Steinman, 1977; Risley, 1968; Sidman, 1953) suggest the availability of procedures for reducing the discriminability of treatment settings and thereby increasing adaptive responding in unsupervised contexts. These findings are important in that they show that desirable behavior need not be restricted to specific discriminative stimuli. As such, they form a basis for extending control to even more distant contingencies.

Delayed Contingencies

As discussed previously, the establishment of generalized and durable adaptive performance is impeded by a reliance on immediate consequences of reinforcement. The delivery of reinforcers and punishers serves as a discriminative stimulus (Koegel & Rincover, 1977) and, as such, predictably distinguishes training

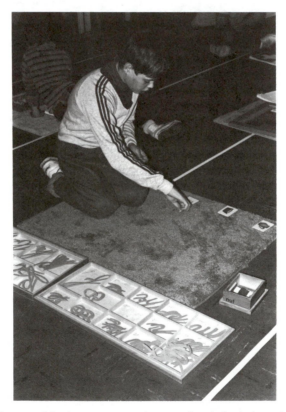

Unpredictable supervision increases on-task responding during independent activities.

from nontraining contexts. Therefore, researchers have explored the use of delayed contingencies to influence behavior that occurs in settings or situations that are not characterized by adequate supervision or reinforcement. While the vast majority of work in this area has been concerned with nonhandicapped or mildly handicapped individuals, there is now sufficient evidence to argue that delayed contingencies can also be used productively with persons who have severe intellectual and behavioral disabilities.

Prior to the 1970s, most of the research on delayed contingencies was conducted with infrahuman subjects within basic research paradigms. The general conclusion derived from this experimental work was that delayed reinforcers slowed the process of response acquisition (Renner, 1964). Subsequent research has included a focus on practical problems of education and behavior management. For example, many investigators have explored the potential of delayed contingencies as a feasible alternative to immediate reinforcement in classroom and other applied settings (e.g., Cousins, Weber, & Dolan, 1984; Ramp, Ulrich, & Dulaney, 1971; Schwartz & Hawkins, 1970). Although the theoretical foundations are not always clear, these applied efforts have demonstrated that relatively remote contingencies can be used productively with many populations and with numerous target behaviors.

Because this chapter is concerned with students with severe handicaps, no attempt is made to review the studies of delayed contingencies with other populations. However, some of the common characteristics of the studies are summarized here. First, virtually all of the studies have been conducted because adequate contingencies could not be provided in the target settings. That is, the procedures were designed to extend the influence of reinforcement to "nontraining" situations. Second, many of the studies have used some kind of feedback or conditioned stimuli to mediate the delay between the target behaviors and the remote contingencies. For example, in efforts to alter the classroom performance of underachieving students, Bailey, Wolf, and Phillips (1970) and Sluyter and Hawkins (1972) used teachers' notes to determine home-based reinforcers. Other researchers have played videotapes (Mayhew & Anderson, 1980; Schwarz & Hawkins, 1970) or audio recordings (Rolider & Van Houten, 1985) of the earlier-occurring target responses when the delayed contingencies were applied. Finally, some of the studies provide evidence that delayed contingencies can facilitate generalization to nontargeted contexts (Fowler & Baer, 1981; Schwarz & Hawkins, 1970). As Stokes and Baer (1977) suggest, the delay of the reinforcement may make it more difficult to detect the limits of the response-reinforcer relationship.

While the delayed contingency techniques seem to offer promise for extending the adaptive responding of developmentally disabled individuals, little research has explicitly addressed this possibility. The following paragraphs review the studies that have been reported. These studies are described in accordance with general behavioral objectives, each of which represents an important concern for the development of increased independence and community functioning.

One major concern pertains to the presence of disruptive responses, such as aggression and tantrums. Displays of these behaviors can restrict community opportunities and may even cause people with severe disabilities to be institutionalized. While tantrums and aggression can often be controlled in training contexts with clear contingencies of reinforcement, their management in nontraining contexts can be much more difficult.

Rolider and Van Houten (1985) described a delayed punishment procedure designed to suppress the public tantrums of children with diverse behavioral and learning disorders. In Rolider and Van Houten's procedure, the tantrums were recorded on a portable tape recorder at the time they occurred. At a later time (e.g., at the end of the day), segments of the tantrums were played to the child and were immediately followed by the administration of a "movement suppression" punishment procedure. Over a series of three experiments, the delayed (and mediated) punishment always produced dramatic reductions of the tantrums.

Delayed contingencies have also been used to control the severe aggressive behavior of a boy and a girl with autism (Dunlap, Johnson, Winterling, & Morelli, in press; Edland & Dunlap, 1984). Both children displayed "situational" aggression; that is, they were never aggressive when they were in the company of some people, but they were highly aggressive with others. The boy ("Fred"), a 12-year-old, only displayed aggression at home with his parents or other family members. The other child, an 8-year-old girl, only displayed aggression toward unfamiliar people, especially young children. The intervention for both children began with immediate, unsignaled contingencies, which were then gradually delayed until an "on-call" system of delayed contingencies could be implemented. The process is illustrated here by a description of Fred's intervention program.

While Fred's behavior was under excellent control at school and with his university-based therapists, his family could not manage his aggressive responses. Even though his parents had been trained to use reinforcement procedures, Fred's aggression had become so severe that an out-of-home placement was threatened. Intervention began by having a therapist (with a remote control listening device) hide in the home and, without warning, provide a stern reprimand immediately following the first aggressive act. Future displays of aggression were similarly treated, but with each additional incident, the time between the aggression and the consequence was extended (and the therapist's presence was never detectable). As the delay was lengthened, from a few seconds to a few minutes and so on, the parents began to inform Fred that they would call his therapist if he acted too aggressively. Thus, immediately following an aggressive act, the victim (parents or siblings) went to the telephone, placed a call, and the therapist would appear on schedule to deliver the reprimand. Throughout the intervention, the therapist also delivered reinforcers on an unpredictable schedule, when instances of appropriate interactions had been displayed. The delay eventually exceeded 2 hours, and the "on-call" system was successful in eliminating Fred's aggression. As shown in Figure 2, the frequency of aggressive acts declined over the course of intervention and, importantly, very intense aggressions were eliminated from the onset of treament. The girl's program was similarly successful and was eventually maintained with contingencies provided by her mother.

The on-call program just described suggests the feasibility of managing the seriously disruptive behavior of severely disabled children with delayed contingencies. However, the generalizability of the results needs to be qualified by noting that: 1) aggression was highly situational, being evident only in certain identifiable contexts; 2) the behavior (aggression) was salient, discrete, and easily detected; 3) the eventual delay was achieved through a gradual fading procedure; and 4) the delayed punisher was consistently mediated by a clear stimulus (i.e., the telephone call), which might not be easy to provide in many public circumstances.

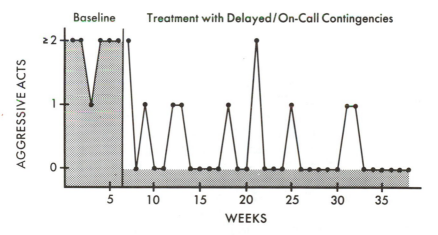

Figure 2. Results of the delayed contingency program for treating "Fred's" aggressive acts in the home setting. Data points reflect the total number of aggressive acts per week, while the shaded portions depict the number of intense aggressive episodes (i.e., those that lasted more than 10 minutes and/or produced physical injury). Data were reported previously by Edlund and Dunlap (1984).

Other concerns pertaining to independent responding by persons with severe handicaps are evident when individuals are placed in normalized classroom or vocational settings. Such environments typically require extended responsive performance without immediate or frequent reinforcement. Unfortunately, many individuals with severe developmental disabilities, such as autism and severe/profound mental retardation, have not learned to respond on the basis of normalized contingencies. While few studies have examined this issue, some investigations are pertinent.

Mayhew and Anderson (1980) reported that two adolescents with severe mental retardation (IQs of 27 and 31) showed improved classroom behavior under conditions of delayed reinforcement. The students' classroom behavior was videotaped. Immediately after the class sessions the tapes were shown, with token reinforcers being provided for appropriate behavior on the tape. While not as effective as immediate reinforcement, the delayed contingency did show improvements over baseline and provided increased resistance to extinction. From a different perspective, Rincover and Koegel (1977) developed procedures for increasing unsupervised task responding by children enrolled in a specialized autism classroom. Their techniques included individualized curricula suitable for independent responding and a systematically fading sequence designed to gradually increase the duration and amount of unsupervised (i.e., unreinforced) responding. The procedures successfully extended the unsupervised responding of even very low functioning autistic children (these procedures are described in detail in Koegel, Rincover, & Russo, 1982).

Dunlap, Koegel, Johnson, and O'Neill (1987) attempted to teach two children with autism to respond on the basis of normalized (i.e., remote) contingencies within integrated classroom settings. A resource specialist implemented a four-component intervention (called STEPS A–D in Figure 3): a) establishing high rates of on-task behavior with frequent rewards and immediate reprimands; b) gradually thinning the schedule of reinforcement; c) gradually establishing and extending the interval (delay) between excess behavior and the contingent reprimand; and d) gradually removing the specialist from the classroom environment. When these steps were completed, the authors implemented a maintenance condition under which contingencies were applied only after every 30 minutes. This condition, labeled "maintenance with post-session contingencies," was designed to resemble a normalized and feasible schedule of explicit teacher supervision, and it was hoped that the four-step training experience would teach the participating children to respond acceptably under such arrangements.

The data for the two 6-year-old autistic children are reproduced in Figure 3. Baseline (BSLN) shows responding without special assistance. The times at which the four training components were initiated are shown by steps A

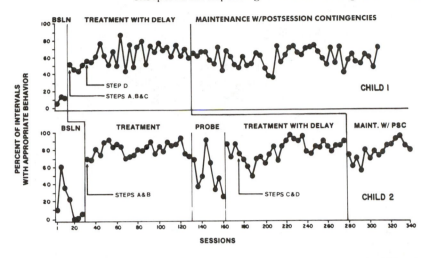

Figure 3. Percentage of intervals with appropriate responding for two autistic children in integrated classroom settings. Data are plotted as blocks of four half-hour sessions. The points at which steps in the treatment process were initiated are labeled as steps A through D (for explanation, see text). (Reprinted with permission from Dunlap, G., Koegel, R.L., Johnson, J., & O'Neill, R.E. [1987]. Maintaining performance of autistic clients in community settings with delayed contingencies. *Journal of Applied Behavior Analysis, 20,* 185–191. Copyright by the Society for the Experimental Analysis of Behavior.)

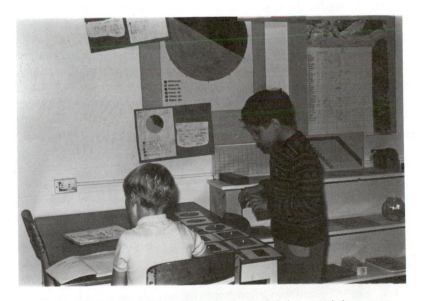

Children with autism can be taught to work independently in integrated classrooms.

through D. The figure shows maintenance under post-session contingencies (PSC) for Child 1. For Child 2, a probe (the same as PSC) introduced prior to the completion of the training progression reveals a failure to maintain. However, when the final two training steps were implemented, maintenance occurred. These procedures and results were also replicated with a young autistic man in a workshop setting (see Dunlap et al., 1987).

In summary, these data demonstrate again the feasibility of teaching individuals with very severe disabilities to respond on the basis of remote, normalized contingencies. They also show, in the case of Child 2, that the teaching may need to be a very gradual process that includes a systematically extended delay of reinforcement, a delay of reprimand, and a very gradual systematic removal of specialized training personnel (cf. Dunlap & Johnson, 1985).

Generalization Effects of Delayed Contingencies

It has been proposed that delayed contingencies may facilitate the generalization of specific training effects (Marholin & Siegel, 1978; Stokes & Baer, 1977). For one thing, the use of delayed consequences has been thought to reduce the discriminability of the training versus nontraining context and thus to facilitate generalization to the nontraining context despite the absence of the training contingencies. Similarly, the delay of reinforcement associated with thinned, intermittent delivery of consequences promotes generalization of responding across the dimension of time, that is, maintenance of responding (Ferster & Skinner, 1957). Training individuals to respond to delayed contingencies may also facilitate the transfer of stimulus control to other contexts.

As previously noted, individuals with severe developmental disabilities can be taught to respond to more remote contingencies by thinning reinforcement schedules and by fading the immediate presence of the trainer. Dunlap, Plienis, and Williams (in press) provided a preliminary analysis of the generalization of unsupervised responding across task activities, trainers, and settings in which a delayed contingency was present, but "untrained." This analysis was conducted with "James," a 20-year-old young adult whose developmental functioning was assessed to be an age equivalent of less than 1½ years. Although ambulatory and self-feeding, James was largely dependent on assistance from family members and caregivers for all other daily life routines.

The primary training task in this investigation consisted of picking up a scattered pile of 67 booklets and putting them in a box. The data in Figure 4 demonstrate that James was capable of performing this "Books" task when the trainer was present in the room and delivering rewards on a continuous reinforcement schedule (CRF). In the next condition (PSC), the trainer delivered the task instruction and then left the room for the duration of the session, asking James to work without immediate supervision for a postsession contingency.

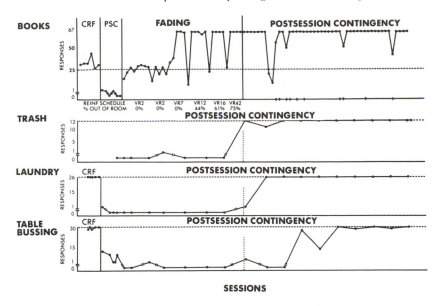

Figure 4.   Training and generalization results for the four tasks throughout the investigation. Total responses completed are shown on the ordinate and sessions are shown on the abscissa. The dashed horizontal lines depict levels of criterion performance. Below the abscissa, the fading progression for the training task is illustrated with the daily averages of the reinforcement schedule and the percent of the session that the trainer was out of the room. Diamonds on the abscissa during PSC indicate those sessions when a brief within-session intervention was provided for the books task. (Reprinted with permission from Dunlap, G., Plienis, A.J., & Williams, L. [in press]. Acquisition and generalization of unsupervised responding: A descriptive analysis. *Journal of The Association for Persons with Severe Handicaps.*)

That is, if James achieved a criterion level of performance, indicated in the figure by the dashed horizontal line, he would earn a reward. During the first PSC condition, James exhibited an almost total absence of responding. In the fading condition, the reinforcement schedule was thinned and the trainer was gradually faded from the room. This eventually produced high and desirable rates of performance when the postsession contingency was reintroduced. In other words, the systematic fading procedure taught James to respond without immediate supervision, and the postsession contingency then served to maintain independent responding over numerous subsequent sessions. (During the second PSC condition with "books," occasional brief interventions were used to increase response rate. These interventions were provided when James did not respond during the first minute of a session and consisted of the trainer reentering the room to provide a verbal prompt ["Do your work"] and/or a brief delivery of the reinforcer. No within-session interventions were ever used during PSC with the other three tasks.)

An additional feature of this investigation was the assessment of three generalization tasks that were systematically probed throughout the study: 1) picking up 12 crumpled pieces of paper and placing them in a trash can ("Trash"); 2) picking up 26 assorted items of clothing and placing them in a laundry basket ("Laundry"); and 3) clearing a table with 6 five-piece place settings ("Table-Bussing"). All probes were conducted with the same post-session contingency that was used in the PSC conditions with "Books." Prior to the completion of the fading condition with "Books," James failed to exhibit any generalization task responses on several consecutive probes. However, at the point at which James successfully completed the fading procedure on "Books" (i.e., when he first completed the entire task without supervision), he also began to respond to all three of the generalized tasks. Unsupervised task completion was immediately evidenced for "Trash," was achieved within two probes for "Laundry," and was soon thereafter exhibited with "Table-Bussing." In other words, generalized unsupervised task responding occurred on all three tasks after James had learned, and continued to maintain, successful responding to the post-session contingency on the "Books" task. Additional generalization probes of all four of these task activities were conducted in naturalistic apartment settings and then with unfamiliar supervisors back at the original training setting. Again, criterion levels of performance were achieved on both of these sets of probes, which assessed additional dimensions of generalization.

The results of this preliminary analysis contain a number of interesting implications. First, they demonstrate the feasibility of teaching individuals with very severe handicaps and long histories of dependency to respond productively without immediate supervision. After a gradual and systematic fading procedure, James learned to maintain responding on the basis of a relatively remote reinforcement contingency. Perhaps more importantly, the training produced generalized effects. This suggests the possibility that the instructional control developed over the course of training generalized across tasks, supervisors, and settings. The implications of such instructional control are, of course, important for the further development of efficient, community-based training protocols.

ISSUES AND FUTURE DIRECTIONS

As illustrated in the previous sections of this chapter, little systematic work has been conducted in which the issue of training individuals with severe handicaps to respond to more remote, delayed contingencies has been emphasized. This concluding section of this chapter summarizes issues that the authors believe are of interest and importance from both theoretical and practical perspectives. It is hoped that this presentation will provide an impetus for further investigation in this area.

The results of Dunlap, Plienis, and Williams (in press) suggest that training unsupervised performance to a delayed contingency facilitates generalization to unsupervised performance on activities with highly similar response requirements. Repetition and extension of this investigation would help to further analyze the dimensions of this effect. Additional analyses of different response requirements, in terms of both the behavioral topography and the effort associated with the task requirement, may prove to be extremely helpful in the development of practical and efficient training procedures to extend independent, unsupervised repertoires of severely handicapped learners. Such analyses may also be beneficial in gaining a better understanding of the transfer of stimulus control in developing generalized performances.

The role of effort as a variable in the acquisition of unsupervised responding to delayed contingencies is also of particular interest. It is reasonable to predict that the probability of completing an unsupervised task will be, in part, a function of the amount of effort associated with the task requirements. For some tasks, a quantification of effort can be assessed as the number of task units required for completion. The authors have collected some pilot data with "Joey," a 4-year-old autistic boy, engaged in picking up toys scattered on the floor of a playroom and putting these toys on a set of shelves. Joey was first exposed to a supervised CRF condition in which he picked up 20 toys at a rate of 4 to 6 toys per minute. During the first five unsupervised PSC sessions, Joey virtually failed to engage in the task. However, on the sixth and subsequent four sessions in this condition, Joey engaged in high rates of responding (10 to 16 toys per minute) and quickly completed the task. The third condition provided a manipulation of the effort variable by placing 70 rather than 20 toys on the floor. The first session of PSC-70 resulted in a high rate of responding and task completion within a time criteria adjusted for the increased number of toys. The subsequent sessions in this condition resulted in a progressive decrement in performance, with a total absence of responding by the fourth session. Reinstatement of the lower task requirement of 20 toys resulted in a return to high rates of task responding within three sessions. A return to the 70-toy requirement replicated the response decrement effect of the previous PSC-70 condition.

Although one can only speculate from these data, it is reasonable to suspect that a gradual increase in the task requirements from 20 to 70 would have been more likely to produce sustained unsupervised performance with postsession contingencies. Just as the principles of shaping and task analysis guide us in the design of programs to teach specific skills, similar considerations may be extremely helpful in guiding the development of independent performance of more effortful activities. Joey's data and the results of Dunlap, Plienis, and Williams (in press) involved simple repetitive task activity. Future investigations may seek to compare the generalization of more complex skills acquired through programmed instruction and errorless learning procedures in contrast to more teacher directed, trial-and-error procedures. One would suspect that the criterion level of unsupervised performance of skills acquired with few errors and minimal teacher direction may more easily come under the control of delayed contingencies. This speculation has important implications for the design of curricular strategies for severely handicapped learners, and, therefore, clearly merits investigation.

In the context of unsupervised responding for delayed contingencies, the authors have also informally observed complex interrelationships between subject characteristics and the nature of the task. For example, in contrast to Joey's data on putting toys away, the authors also observed him exhibit sustained independent performance on another task despite a large increase in the task requirements. After a brief training sequence, Joey would consistently complete a sorting task involving 10 each of 5 different objects (e.g., blue or red squares, blue or red circles, etc.) for a total of 50 items to be sorted. Increasing both the complexity (10 groups of stimulus items) and the amount of items (200) did not detract from Joey's independent performance. One post hoc account of this performance calls on Joey's notable history of self-initiated perseverative activities, which shared compulsive qualities similar to the required sorting task. This suggests that certain learner characteristics can be matched to task characteristics in promoting unsupervised responding, similar to the matching of vocational skills to client characteristics as discussed by Sailor, Goetz, Anderson, Hunt, and Gee in Chapter 4. However, these observations further underscore the need to investigate how these behavioral predilections can be generalized across a broader spectrum of desirable unsupervised activities under the control of remote contingencies.

Further assessment and analyses of strategies that help mediate temporal delays between behavior and consequences are also desirable. Audio and videotaped recordings have been demonstrated to be effective in this regard (Mayhew & Anderson, 1980; Rolider & Van Houten, 1985). Cognitive perspectives in normal development would suggest that these recordings may serve as a prosthetic adaptation for deficits in imaginal representation and memory processes associated with developmental disabilities. From a behavioral perspective, furture research should further investigate the mediational and conditioned stimulus functions of such strategies. Although explanations may remain speculative within the context of current methodologies, replication and extensions of such procedures may help determine the appropriateness for specific subgroups of learners, and other parameters related to implementation, efficiency, and generalization. It may also prove to be beneficial to combine such mediational strategies with schedule thinning and stimulus fading procedures to facilitate the development of unsupervised responding for some individuals.

SUMMARY AND CONCLUSION

In summary, achieving higher levels of independent responding in the repertoires of severely handicapped learners is an integral objective, implicitly or explicitly, directly or indirectly, across all treatment and training procedures. Although our ability to increase the behavioral repertoires of handicapped learners has greatly expanded, many individuals with severe handicaps fail to exhibit generalization of newly acquired skills beyond the training conditions. These training conditions often include close supervision by relatively skilled trainers who typically deliver frequent immediate consequences. Although one way to address these concerns is through the development of self-management strategies, this chapter has attempted to provide a systematic framework for an alternative approach to the problem. This alternative is the development and analysis of procedures to train unsupervised responding to more remote contingencies. Although this is a rather obvious extension of well-documented training principles and procedures, little exploration of this approach has been reported.

Some evidence has been offered to suggest that the failure to respond to a broader range of delayed contingencies may reflect a critical, if not a keystone, deficit for some severely handicapped learners. The deficit undoubtedly impedes much community integration and can be related to organismic as well as environmental-historical factors. Importantly, data are beginning to suggest that the deficiency can be overcome through direct, systematic training procedures.

In recent years, a trend in behavior analysis and special education has been to focus on pivotal responses and skill areas that may impact broadly and generatively on the life-styles of persons with severe disabilities (e.g., Evans & Meyer, 1985; Guess & Siegel-Causey, 1985). An important aspect of this emphasis is the development of increased independence, self-reliance, and the ability to respond adaptively in the absence of specialized supervision (Shevin & Klein, 1984). While many curricular and programmatic directions may contribute to this critical objective, the role of remote contingencies is likely to be a pervasive influence, a factor that can improve the efficiency and generalized efficacy of our training efforts.

REFERENCES

Bailey, J.S., Wolf, M.M., & Phillips, E.L. (1970). Home-based reinforcement and the modification of pre-delinquents' classroom behavior. *Journal of Applied Behavior Analysis, 3,* 223–233.

Browder, D.M., & Shapiro, E.S. (1985). Applications of self-management to individuals with severe handicaps. *Journal of The Association for Persons with Severe Handicaps, 10,* 200–208.

Corte, H.E., Wolf, M.M., & Locke, B.J. (1971). A comparison of procedures for eliminating self-injurious behavior of retarded adolescents. *Journal of Applied Behavior
Analysis, 4,* 201–214.

Cousins, L.S., Weber, E.M., & Dolan, K. (1984). *"How long do I have to stay after
school?" Delayed punishment effects in and out of the classroom.* Paper presented at
the 18th Annual Convention of the Association for the Advancement of Behavior
Therapy, Philadelphia.

Drabman, R.S., Hammer, D., & Rosenbaum, M.S. (1979). Assessing generalization in
behavior modification with children: The generalization map. *Behavioral Assessment, 1,* 203–219.

Dunlap, G., & Johnson, J. (1985). Increasing the independent responding of autistic
children with unpredictable supervision. *Journal of Applied Behavior Analysis, 18,*
227–236.

Dunlap, G., Johnson, J., Winterling, V., & Morelli, M. (in press). The management of
disruptive behavior in unsupervised settings: Issues and directions for a behavioral
technology. *Education and Treatment of Children.*

Dunlap, G., Koegel, R.L., & Burke, J.C. (1981). Educational implications of stimulus
overselectivity in autistic children. *Exceptional Education Quarterly, 2,* 37–49.

Dunlap, G., Koegel, R.L., Johnson, J., & O'Neill, R.E. (1987). Maintaining performance of autistic clients in community settings with delayed contingencies. *Journal
of Applied Behavior Analysis, 20,* 185–191.

Dunlap, G., Plienis, A.J., & Williams, L. (in press). Acquisition and generalization of
unsupervised responding: A descriptive analysis. *Journal of the Association for Persons with Severe Handicaps.*

Edland, C., & Dunlap, G. (1984, May). *Controlling situational aggression with delayed
contingencies.* Paper presented at the Sixth Annual Conference on Behavior Analysis
and Therapy, Camarillo, CA.

Egel, A.L. (1982). Generalization and maintenance. In R.L. Koegel, A. Rincover, &
A.L. Egel (Eds.) *Educating and understanding autistic children* (pp. 281–300). San
Diego: College-Hill Press.

Evans, I.M., & Meyer, L.H. (1985). *An educative approach to behavior problems: A
practical decision model for interventions with severely handicapped learners.* Baltimore: Paul H. Brookes Publishing Co.

Ferster, C.B., & Skinner, B.F. (1957). *Schedules of reinforcement.* New York: Appleton-
Century-Crofts.

Fowler, S., & Baer, D.M. (1981). "Do I have to be good all day?" The timing of delayed
reinforcement as a factor in generalization. *Journal of Applied Behavior Analysis, 14,*
13–24.

Fowler, S.A., Baer, D.M., & Stolz, S.B. (Eds.). (1984). Self management tactics for
the developmentally disabled [Special issue]. *Analysis and Intervention in Developmental Disabilities, 4*(2).

Guess, D., & Siegel-Causey, E. (1985). Behavioral control and education of severely
handicapped students: Who's doing what to whom? and why? In D. Bricker & J. Filler
(Eds.), *Severe mental retardation: From theory to practice* (pp. 230–244). Reston,
VA: Council for Exceptional Children.

Horner, R.H., Bellamy, G.T., & Colvin, G.T. (1984). Responding in the presence of
non-trained stimuli: Implications of generalization error patterns. *Journal of The Association for Persons with Severe Handicaps, 9,* 287–295.

Horner, R.H., Meyer, L.H., & Fredericks, H.D.B. (Eds.). (1986). *Education of learners with severe handicaps: Exemplary service strategies.* Baltimore: Paul H. Brookes Publishing Co.

Koegel, R.L., & Covert, A. (1972). The relationship of self-stimulation to learning in autistic children. *Journal of Applied Behavior Analysis, 5,* 381–388.

Koegel, R.L., & Rincover, A. (1977). Research on the difference between generalization and maintenance in extra-therapy settings. *Journal of Applied Behavior Analysis, 10,* 1–12.

Koegel, R.L., Rincover, A., & Egel, A.L. (Eds.). (1982). *Educating and understanding autistic children.* San Diego: College-Hill Press.

Koegel, R.L., Rincover, A., & Russo, D.C. (1982). Classroom management: Progression from special to normal classrooms. In R.L. Koegel, A. Rincover, & A.L. Egel (Eds.), *Educating and understanding autistic children* (pp. 203–241). San Diego: College-Hill Press.

Koegel, R.L., Schreibman, L., Johnson, J., O'Neill, R.E., & Dunlap, G. (1984). Collateral effects of parent training on families with autistic children. In R. Dangel & R. Polster (Eds.), *Behavioral parent training: Issues in research and practice* (pp. 358–378). New York: Guilford Press.

Liberty, K.A. (1984). Self-monitoring and skill generalization: A review of current research. In M. Boer (Ed.), *Investigating the problem of skill generalization: Literature review I* (pp. 37–53). Institute for the Education of Severely Handicapped Children, Washington Research Organization. (U.S. Department of Education, Contract No. 300-82-0364). Seattle: University of Washington, College of Education.

Lovaas, O.I. (1977). *The autistic child: Language development through behavior modification.* New York: Irvington.

Lovaas, O.I., Koegel, R.L., & Schreibman, L. (1979). Stimulus overselectivity in autism: A review of research. *Psychological Bulletin, 86,* 1236–1254.

Lovaas, O.I., & Newsom, C.D. (1976). Behavior modification with psychotic children. In H. Leitenberg (Ed.), *Handbook of behavior modification and behavior therapy* (pp. 303–360). Englewood Cliffs, NJ: Prentice-Hall.

Marholin, D., & Siegel, L.J. (1978). Beyond the law of effect: Programming for the maintenance of behavioral change. In D. Marholin (Ed.), *Child behavior therapy.* New York: Gardner Press.

Marholin, D., & Steinman, W.M. (1977). Stimulus control in the classroom as a function of the behavior reinforced. *Journal of Applied Behavior Analysis, 10,* 456–478.

Mayhew, G.L., & Anderson, J. (1980). Delayed and immediate reinforcement: Retarded adolescents in an educational setting. *Behavior Modification, 4,* 527–545.

Paine, S.C., Radicchi, J., Rosellini, L.C., Deutchman, L., & Darch, C. (1983). *Structuring your classroom for academic success.* Champaign, IL: Research Press.

Ramp, E., Ulrich, R., & Dulaney, S. (1971). Delayed timeout as a procedure for reducing disruptive classroom behaviors: A case study. *Journal of Applied Behavior Analysis, 4,* 235–239.

Renner, K.E. (1964). Delay of reinforcement: A historical review. *Psychological Bulletin, 61,* 341–361.

Rincover, A., & Koegel, R.L. (1977). Classroom treatment of autistic children: II. Individualized instruction in a group. *Journal of Abnormal Child Psychology, 5,* 113–126.

Risley, T.R. (1968). The effects and side effects of punishing the autistic behaviors of a deviant child. *Journal of Applied Behavior Analysis, 1,* 21–34.

Rolider, A., & Van Houten, R. (1985). Suppressing tantrum behavior in public places through the use of delayed punishment mediated by audio recordings. *Behavior Therapy, 16,* 181–194.

Schwarz, M.L., & Hawkins, R.P. (1970). Application of delayed reinforcement procedures to the behavior of an elementary school child. *Journal of Applied Behavior Analysis, 3,* 85–96.

Shevin, M., & Klein, N.K. (1984). The importance of choice-making skills for students with severe disabilities. *Journal of The Association for Persons with Severe Handicaps, 9,* 159–166.

Sidman, M. (1953). Avoidance conditioning with brief shock and no exteroceptive warning signal. *Science, 118,* 157–158.

Skinner, B.F. (1968). *The technology of teaching.* Englewood Cliffs, NJ: Prentice-Hall.

Sluyter, D.J., & Hawkins, R.P. (1972). Delayed reinforcement of classroom behavior by parents. *Journal of Learning Disabilities, 5,* 20–28.

Stokes, T.F., & Baer, D.M. (1977). An implicit technology of generalization. *Journal of Applied Behavior Analysis, 10,* 349–368.

Stokes, T.F., & Osnes, P.G. (1986). Programming the generalization of children's social behavior. In P.S. Strain, M.J. Guralnick, & H. Walker (Eds.), *Children's social behavior: Development, assessment, and modification* (pp. 407–443). Orlando, FL: Academic Press.

Van Houten, R. (1986, May). *Right of clients to effective treatment.* Paper presented at the 12th annual convention of the Association for Behavior Analysis, Milwaukee.

Chapter 7 ――――――――――――

The Effects of Peer-Mediated Interventions on Establishing, Maintaining, and Generalizing Children's Behavior Changes

Susan A. Fowler

Children as students in classrooms sometimes play dual roles. In addition to being students, teammates, and followers, they sometimes are teachers, leaders, captains, and monitors. Their assistantship and management roles can be an integral part of an effective and efficiently conducted classroom. This chapter discusses the characteristics of classroom interventions for children that are mediated by children. The focus is on interventions designed to reduce problem behaviors such as aggression, negative interactions, nonparticipation, and off-task performance. The role of children in these interventions as both the provider of the intervention (e.g., peer-monitor, team captain, manager) and the recipient of the intervention is examined.

Thus far, research has demonstrated that peer-mediated interventions are effective in changing the social behaviors of children receiving the intervention. In fact, several recent studies suggest that interventions mediated by peers are comparable in their effects to interventions implemented by adults (e.g., Carden-Smith & Fowler, 1984; Phillips, Phillips, Wolf, & Fixsen, 1973). For instance, children can be trained to teach other children with social deficiencies appropriate social initiations and responses (e.g., Goldstein & Wickstrom, 1986; Odom & Strain, 1986; Strain, 1983), offers to share (Kohler & Fowler, 1985), and affection behaviors (e.g., Twardosz, Nordquist, Simon, & Botkin, 1983). Likewise, they also can be trained to monitor and modify peers' rates of appropriate participation in classroom activities (e.g., Drabman, 1973; Greenwood, Sloane, & Baskin, 1974).

The use of peers as intervention agents has great appeal, for several reasons. Peers are often readily available, and as such represent a natural resource as intervention agents. Perhaps most importantly, they actively affect one another's behavior. Charlesworth and Hartup (1967) demonstrated a positive correlation between the number of positive behaviors that children directed to peers and received from peers; they demonstrated a similar relationship with negative behaviors. Their data suggest the interdependency of children's behavior: the social behaviors of one child are influenced by the social behaviors of other children.

The interdependent nature of children's social behavior provides a strong rationale for providing active roles to peers in interventions with children. It should be pointed out that children, albeit intentionally or not, may contribute to another child's undesirable behaviors (e.g., aggression) or social deficits (e.g., lack of initiations). The following examples represent four ways that children may support undesirable behavior.

1. Peers may support inappropriate behavior by actively reinforcing it. For instance, Solomon and Wahler (1973) demonstrated in an elementary classroom that attention from classmates maintained the disruptive behavior of five students in the class; withdrawal of the classmates' attention subsequently resulted in a reduction of disruption.
2. Peers may support some inappropriate behavior through negative reinforcement. Patterson and his colleagues have speculated that one child's aggression may be reinforced by another child's acquiescence to the aggressive episode (e.g., Patterson, Littman, & Bricker, 1976). In this example, a child's use of verbal taunts and physical threats may be maintained by peers who give in to the threats (e.g., by relinquishing toys) in order to escape the threats and avoid a probable fight.
3. In yet other instances, children may ignore and fail to reinforce appropriate overtures from peers, thus extinguishing desirable new responses from them. Hendrickson, Strain, Tremblay, and Shores (1982) demonstrated

that handicapped children often failed to respond to initiations from other children.
4. And, in a few instances, peers may actively punish appropriate responses from a peer. They may refuse social initiations or offers.

These four factors suggest that peers sometimes may need explicit training in how to respond (and not respond) to a child's new behavior or behavior change during and after intervention. In these cases, peers may need to learn to attend to certain appropriate behaviors instead of to former, inappropriate behaviors. Or, they may need to learn that interactions with a child can be pleasant and safe and not threatening or negative. Likewise, they may need to learn to respond affirmatively to initiations from a usually withdrawn child.

Alternatively, the new behaviors acquired by some children during intervention may change their peers' behavior with little or no training required for the peers. For example, Kohler and Fowler (1985) taught three socially deficient youngsters to verbalize offers to share with classmates; the classmates of two of the children immediately and spontaneously reciprocated with additional offers to share. After training was withdrawn, the cycle of reciprocated offers continued; the two children who were no longer socially deficient continued to share, and their peers continued to reciprocate with new offers to share. The peers of the third child, however, required direct intervention, in the form of prompts to share and external contingencies for sharing, before they reliably reciprocated her offers.

Researchers have argued that peers can provide support not only for maintaining behavior changes, as demonstrated by Kohler and Fowler (1985), but also for generalizing behavior changes to a variety of settings and activities in which intervention is unlikely to occur owing to cost, accessibility, convenience, or a variety of other factors. Unfortunately, the extent to which peer-mediated interventions promote generalized and enduring changes beyond the intervention time and setting has not been consistently demonstrated, and often has not been investigated. Additional research is necessary to determine the conditions under which and ways in which peers may facilitate maintenance and generalization of change.

This chapter discusses three ways for involving peers in interventions designed to reduce problem behaviors such as negative interactions or disruption. The role that peers play in these interventions as both therapist and client is discussed. In most interventions involving peers as change agents, children's appointments to supervisory or teaching roles have been based on merit or skill. These children frequently are either older, better behaved, or better accomplished than the children whom they assist (e.g., Egel, Richman, & Koegel, 1981; Lancioni, 1982; Schreibman, O'Neill, & Koegel, 1983). However, the intervention programs presented in this chapter suggest that such skills or attributions may not always be necessary. Recent research suggests that children in need of direct intervention can be taught to supervise or tutor their peers in the very behaviors or skills that they themselves often fail to exhibit (e.g., Drabman, 1973; Fowler, Dougherty, Kirby, & Kohler, 1986).

THREE MODELS OF PEER-MEDIATED INTERVENTIONS

Research conducted by this author and her colleagues suggests that peer-mediated interventions can be introduced in three ways. The first model follows the most traditional approach by placing the child who has the undesirable behaviors in the role of client. This child then typically receives an intervention mediated by another child, often a classmate. Selection of the peer mediator is usually based on demonstration of exemplary social skills, popularity, and history of compliance with teacher instructions. One child may serve as a therapist, or a small pool of children may be appointed to the role, with members of the pool rotating appointments as therapists across days. This model has most frequently been used within the social skills training literature (e.g., Egel et al., 1981; Strain, Kerr, & Ragland, 1981). For purposes of clarity, this model will be termed here the "subject as client model."

A second model rotates the assignment of peer therapist across all members of a group. In this model, some members of the group may be in need of intervention and treatment, whereas other members of the group are not. Children take turns assuming the roles of therapist and client. Appointment to the role of therapist may be contingent on the child's demonstrating a criterion level of acceptable behavior. In these cases, the appointment serves as a reward for improved performance. This model will be referred to as the "subject alternating as client and therapist model."

A third model involves the appointment of the child in need of intervention to the role of therapist. In this model, the child who is in need of intervention serves as a peer therapist to one or more classmates. Instead of receiving points for improved performance, the child awards points to designated classmates when they engage in exemplary behavior. The intent of this model is: 1) to provide children with new patterns of positive interaction, albeit somewhat artificial, which may replace their former patterns of negative or coercive interaction and 2) to promote imitative learning by focusing the child's attention on the desirable behaviors that the child is asked to monitor. This case will be referred to here as the "subject as therapist model."

Examples of each of these three models follow, along with a discussion of the advantages and disadvantages of each model. First, however, each model is discussed according to features identified as common to most peer-mediated programs; these features are presented in Table 1 and discussed next.

Table 1.   Features common to most peer-mediated programs

1.   Criteria for participation:
    a.   Selection of children to be monitors
    b.   Selection of children to be monitored
2.   Rules for participation:
    a.   For the behaviors that are to be peer-monitored
    b.   For the peer-monitoring system
3.   Reward systems:
    a.   For the monitored child
    b.   For the monitor
4.   Training:
    a.   Role-plays
    b.   Transfer of the monitoring strategy to the classroom activity for which it was designed
    c.   Adult supervision of the monitoring system
    d.   Gradual reduction of adult supervision
5.   Assessment of effects:
    a.   Consumer satisfaction surveys
    b.   Assessment of treatment effect
    c.   Assessment of treatment maintenance
    d.   Assessment of the monitored child's generalized behavior changes
    e.   Assessment of the peer-monitor's generalized behavior changes

GUIDELINES FOR DEVELOPING A PEER-MEDIATED INTERVENTION

Criteria for Participation in the Intervention

Criteria for selection of children to serve as the peer therapist should be considered prior to the onset of any program. However, the criteria may vary, depending on the model selected. For example, children who are compliant with adult instructions, who are reliable school attenders, and who display the behaviors targeted for intervention at acceptable rates usually have been selected to serve as peer monitors. Yet, these characteristics may not be vital to the success of the intervention. Selection should depend on the training and supervision provided to the monitor, the reward system used, and the goals of the intervention. If extensive training and supervision are provided, then children with fewer skills and lower rates of acceptable behavior can also serve as monitors.

Likewise, criteria for selection of the children who participate as clients in the peer-mediated intervention will vary, depending on the model. In the traditional subject as client model, children most in need of intervention are selected to be clients. The opposite may be true for the other two models. For instance, children capable of modeling good behavior may serve, at least some of the time, as the client in models in which the child most in need of intervention serves as the therapist or alternates as therapist. The participation of children with exemplary behavior as clients provides opportunities for the child designated as therapist to interact with skilled peers and to observe and provide consequences for skilled behavior.

Rules for Participation

Most intervention programs contain rules governing the behaviors (e.g., social isolation, noncompliance) that have been targeted for intervention. In interventions conducted by children, such rules should be few in number and simple in form (e.g., stay on the playground, find a partner, take turns with the soccer ball), so that both child-therapist and client can remember them. Both the children who implement the intervention and those who receive the intervention should be able to state the rules and identify examples of compliance and noncompliance with the rules. Obviously, children able to identify the rules will be more likely to provide appropriate consequences for rule following or rule infractions. Teaching a few simple rules may also facilitate generalization to other times or settings in which the rules are applicable.

In peer-mediated interventions, rules also will be needed for the children conducting the intervention. The purpose of these rules should be to ensure that the intervention program is administered in a positive and equitable manner. For instance, such rules may guide the use of a point system and indicate how to resolve a dispute between therapist and client. Peer intervention programs also should contain guidelines or rules for when a peer-therapist should seek adult assistance or intervention.

Development of a Reward System

Peer-mediated interventions often contain a simple point or check mark system in which peer therapists recognize desirable behaviors by awarding a point or check mark. In some cases, peer therapists recognize undesirable performance by withholding point awards. Point awards or totals then may be posted and/or exchanged for tangible rewards. The criterion for a reward is based on the number of points or checks earned. The author and her colleagues have set the criterion at less than 100% of the available points; for instance, criterion might be reached with three out of four points. This criterion guarantees that children can receive feedback from the monitor regarding low rates of unacceptable behavior, without losing their reward. Bonus incentives may be provided for earning all available points.

The author and her colleagues have introduced a point system in interventions for several reasons: 1) often young children are not comfortable, skilled, or effective at spontaneously praising one another's behavior (e.g., Warren, Baer, & Rogers-Warren, 1979); 2) point awards provide a clear message that children have behaved appropriately (e.g., Kazdin, 1977); and 3) points that are awarded by peers and later exchanged for a tangible reward appear to be stronger reinforcers than peer praise, at least initially.

In some cases the reward systems have contained a group contingency. That is, the reward earned by the children who receive points is provided to all members of the class. For instance, the monitored children may exchange their points at the end of the week for their entire class to view a filmstrip or take a brief field trip. In other cases, rewards have been available only to the children earning the points. Group contingencies often are used to increase classmates' cooperation with or support for the monitoring procedure (cf. Greenwood & Hops, 1981).

Training

Training may be provided throughout much of the peer-mediated intervention. Three levels of training are recommended. First, role-plays may be used to introduce children to the program and to teach the basic roles and rules of therapist and client. During the role-play, children rehearse the rules, practice the intervention strategy, and practice the desirable targeted behaviors. An adult provides consistent and contingent feedback regarding the children's use of the intervention strategy and performance of the targeted behavior. Adult prompts and feedback are reduced gradually during practice, as children demonstrate competency in implementing the intervention strategy and participating in the intervention.

Transfer of the monitoring strategy to the classroom activity for which it was designed is the next step of training. Adult supervision should be provided, at least initially, to ensure that the program works as intended. Supervision includes providing corrective feedback to the therapists regarding their point awards. The provision of corrective feedback during the initial sessions of a peer-mediated intervention can assist children in further differentiating acceptable behaviors from unacceptable behaviors. For instance, therapists initially may award or withhold some points inaccurately. Their inaccurate point awards may reflect faulty discrimination regarding the acceptability of a behavior. Or, if points are awarded only at the end of an activity, their errors may be due to forgetfulness regarding an earlier event. Reluctance or failure to withhold a point, however, may reflect also a child's discomfort at penalizing a peer for inappropriate behavior. These errors can be guarded against by having an adult supervise, and when necessary correct, point awards and withholdings. So far, reports of unmerited point fines or withholdings in the child peer-monitoring literature have been rare (cf. Fowler, 1986).

The last phase of training involves gradual reduction of adult supervision, until it is finally withdrawn, or at least becomes intermittent and unpredictable.

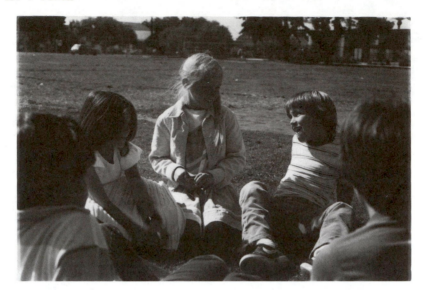

Peer monitoring can be used to maintain and sometimes even to establish behavior change. In this photo, the children have been taught to monitor each other's behavior during recess, following gradual withdrawal of adult supervision.

The ability of children to participate in the program under reduced levels of supervision will dictate the extent to which adult support is withdrawn.

Assessment

Several forms of assessment should be conducted to determine the direct and indirect effects produced by the peer-mediated interventions and the likelihood that the intervention has produced enduring and generalized behavior changes. The following assessment procedures should be considered:

1. Consumer satisfaction surveys may be used to determine the extent to which children like the peer-monitoring intervention. These surveys may be given both to children who serve as therapists as well as to children who serve as clients. They are used to assess children's satisfaction with the point procedure, with the reward system, and with their intervention roles (client or therapist).
2. Assessments of the intervention's effectiveness should be conducted on a daily basis to ensure that the procedures are working and are being implemented properly. Such assessments should examine both the client's and therapist's behavior, as well as the rate (or availability) of adult supervision. If the intervention is not producing consistent and desirable results, the role of the therapist should be examined carefully to determine if the

therapist is implementing the intervention accurately. Peer-mediated interventions can and should be interrupted or replaced with an adult-implemented intervention, if effects produced during the peer-mediated intervention are not satisfactory.

3. Maintenance of behavior changes should be assessed at least occasionally to determine if continued intervention is needed. Such assessment may be conducted by suspending the intervention for several days or a week.

4. Likewise, the extent to which the child as client generalizes behavior changes produced during the intervention should be assessed whenever possible, by collecting data during similar activities in which no intervention is conducted. One reason cited for the use of peer-mediated interventions has been that children may facilitate generalization both passively and actively. Perhaps the client will generalize the targeted behaviors to other activities, when children involved in the intervention are present in these activities (e.g., Stokes & Baer, 1976). If not, these same children may actively recruit the client to exhibit the behaviors targeted in intervention (e.g., Johnston & Johnston, 1972).

5. Finally, the extent to which the children who serve as clients generalize changes in their behavior also merits assessment. Such assessments should examine: 1) if therapists generalize their prompts and praise to peers and 2) if therapists show changes in the very behaviors they are monitoring in other children (e.g., rate of positive peer interactions).

EXAMPLES OF PEER-MEDIATED INTERVENTIONS

The author and her colleagues have conducted a series of studies illustrating the three models of peer-mediated intervention. In these studies, children have been appointed to monitor one another for disruptive, aggressive, or noncompliant behavior. The purpose of the interventions has been to increase cooperative peer interactions or to increase participation in class routines. Children who participated in these interventions have ranged in ability level; interventions have included children achieving within the normal range, children with developmental delays, children with mild to moderate retardation, and children exhibiting behavior disorders. The age of participating children has ranged from 5 years to 11 years. Three of these studies are described here to illustrate the three models of peer-mediated interventions.

The Subject as Client Model

A study conducted by Dougherty, Fowler, and Paine (1985) illustrates the more traditional form of peer-mediated intervention. In this study, the primary subject, named Dennis, received intervention from classmates, whose behavior was somewhat better than Dennis's behavior. Dennis and his classmates were enrolled in a special education class for students diagnosed as mildly or moderately retarded and who ranged in age from 8 to 10 years. The peer-monitoring model was implemented during daily recess, with the goals of decreasing Dennis's negative peer interactions and rule infractions and increasing his positive peer interactions. The monitoring system that we used was adapted from the R.E.C.E.S.S. program developed by Hill Walker and his colleagues in Oregon (cf. Walker et al., 1978) The R.E.C.E.S.S. program was designed for adult implementation; as such Dougherty et al. (1985) preceded the peer-monitoring condition with a condition initially implemented by adults. Following a demonstration that monitoring by adults could change Dennis's behavior effectively, peers were appointed to manage the monitoring system. The following procedures were used during the peer-monitoring phases.

Criteria for Participation Six classmates were selected to take turns as monitors for Dennis. The children were chosen on the basis of positive teacher ratings, peer ratings, and screening observations. Dennis was selected to be monitored based on his very high rates of negative peer interactions (1.0–2.0 per minute). Because Dennis's behavior appeared volatile, the initial peer-monitoring condition was preceded by adult-monitoring conditions, in which Dougherty et al. (1985) first reduced his negative behavior.

Rules for Participation Thirteen playground rules were introduced and rehearsed with all members of the class prior to adult monitoring. These rules were posted in the classroom and were reviewed frequently during the peer-monitoring condition. Likewise, rules for the peer monitor were developed. Peer monitors were instructed to: 1) model appropriate behavior during recess, with an emphasis on interacting positively with peers, 2) remind Dennis to follow playground rules and play with his classmates, 3) award Dennis a point when he played with peers and when he avoided a negative interaction, and 4) fine Dennis a point when he broke a rule or fought. An additional rule was developed for Dennis in his role as the monitored child. The rule stated that Dennis would be fined an extra point if he argued with his monitor regarding a point fine.

Reward Systems The original R.E.C.E.S.S. point system was used. Dennis began each recess with four points, which his monitor could subtract one at a time for negative behavior. He also had the opportunity to earn two bonus points for good behavior, which could not be subtracted from his total. Points were exchanged daily after recess for a small-group activity (such as bingo or map reading), which Dennis shared with his peer monitor and another classmate. Points also were accumulated for a class reward (e.g., filmstrip viewing, extra recess time), which was available at the end of each week that Dennis earned the criterion number of points. All members of the class participated in this activity. The group reward was introduced to encourage all members of the class to help Dennis keep points and earn points.

Training Dennis and the peer-monitors role-played examples of positive interactions and negative interactions with an adult. In addition, they identified rule infractions from vignettes presented by the adult. They also rehearsed giving and receiving point awards and point fines. Training required approximately 2 hours. After training was completed, the peer-monitoring intervention was implemented in the morning recess; several weeks later, it was extended to the afternoon recess. Dennis was monitored daily in both recesses by a peer. One peer monitor was assigned per recess; students rotated their appointments across the group.

An adult was present on the playground to prompt the peer monitor to watch Dennis and to award or withdraw a point when appropriate. The adult also was available to intervene if Dennis argued with his monitor regarding a point fine. Such arguments were rare, since they resulted in an automatic point fine for Dennis. The adult supervisor gradually reduced her prompts to the monitors over the course of several weeks and finally ceased all prompting. The supervisor continued to praise Dennis—typically once or twice every recess—for his appropriate behavior.

Assessments Consumer satisfaction surveys and direct observations were collected throughout this study. Consumer satisfaction surveys were administered to Dennis and to the six classmates who monitored him. Children appointed as monitors consistently rated their monitoring tasks as "very much liked," with the exception of point fines, which were "not liked." In fact, peer monitors used point fines infrequently; Dennis lost a total of 18 points in 116 peer-monitored recesses. Likewise, Dennis rated his role as client in the monitoring relationship as "very much liked." Interestingly, near the end of the study, Dennis was asked to monitor a classmate during the noon recess and initially objected, stating that he preferred to be monitored.

Daily observations were conducted to assess the effects of the intervention on Dennis's behavior. These data are presented in Figure 1. During the morning recess, Dennis's negative interactions were reduced initially by an adult monitoring condition, which was implemented first by one of the experimenters (i.e., a consultant) and then by Dennis's classroom teachers. These improvements were maintained throughout the extended peer-monitoring condition. Although not presented in Figure 1, Dennis's rate of positive interaction also increased, simultaneous with the decrease in negative interaction. Peer monitoring subsequently was introduced to the afternoon recess; here again, the procedure effectively reduced Dennis's negative behavior. Near the end of

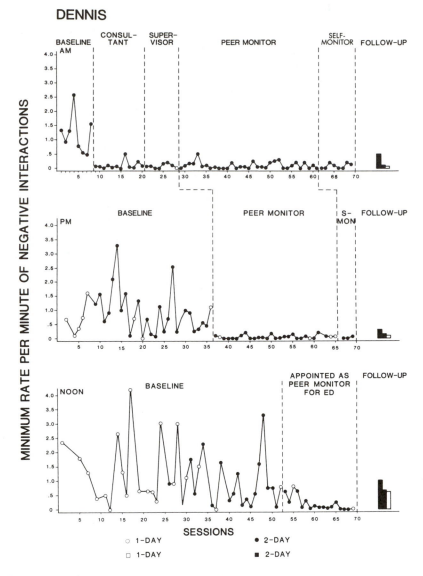

Figure 1. Minimum rate per minute of negative interactions by Dennis during the three daily recesses (see discussion in text). (Reprinted with permission from Dougherty, B.S., Fowler, S.A., & Paine, S. [1985]. The use of peer monitors to reduce negative interactions during recess. *Journal of Applied Behavior Analysis, 18,* 141–153.)

the study (and the school year), brief self-monitoring conditions were implemented in both morning and afternoon recess, where again the positive behavior changes were maintained.

Intervention effects were assessed the following school year, 3 months after all intervention ended, to determine maintenance of the behavior change. Dennis's rate of negative interactions remained well below his original baseline levels; on the 5 days sampled, his rate ranged from the low rate established during intervention to rates slightly higher than intervention. His rate of positive interaction remained high.

Generalization assessments were conducted by introducing the second peer-monitoring condition to the afternoon recess in a delayed fashion and by withholding intervention from the noon recess for an extended number of weeks. Dennis did not generalize improvements maintained or established during peer monitoring in the morning recess to either the afternoon or the noon recess; his rate of negative interactions remained high in both recesses until interventions were introduced.

An interesting generalized change was noted in the behavior of Dennis's peers. Negative interactions from peers to Dennis decreased substantially in each setting, following the introduction of an intervention in that setting. These low rates were maintained through the end of the school year.

Finally, the peer-monitors' behavior was assessed frequently to determine if their involvement in the intervention produced positive or negative changes in their behavior on the playground both during and outside of intervention sessions. Four peer monitors who exhibited undesirable rates of negative interactions decreased these rates in the morning and afternoon recess during their appointment as monitors. Furthermore, they maintained these improvements during the peer-monitoring condition even on days in which they were not appointed to be monitors.

In summary, the subject as client model for peer monitoring can be a very effective procedure for maintaining reductions, established through adult-monitoring. The results of this study also suggest that peer-monitoring can be used to extend behavior change to previously untreated time periods or settings of the day. Observations of the monitors suggest, too, that they may benefit from their appointment role by modifying their own negative interactions. Satisfaction data collected during the study indicated that the monitors enjoyed their role of monitoring, although they did *not* like to withdraw points. Likewise, Dennis reported that he enjoyed being monitored by peers.

The Subject Alternating as Client and Therapist Model

A study conducted by Carden-Smith and Fowler (1984) serves to illustrate the subject alternating as client and therapist model. Carden-Smith and Fowler examined the effectiveness of a peer-monitored token system on reducing disruptive behavior and nonparticipation during a daily classroom transition period in two summer session kindergartens. The transition period included three activities: classroom cleanup, bathrooming, and waiting for a large group activity. Each classroom was made up of nine children referred to the program for serious behavior and/or learning problems. The peer-monitoring procedure involved the assignment of children to teams and the daily appointment of children as team captains or monitors. All children in each classroom participated in the intervention. The following procedures were used.

Criteria for Participation All children eventually took turns as team captains/peer monitors. Eligibility for the appointment as team captain was established daily and was based on the appointed child exhibiting a criterion level of appropriate behavior during the preceding day. Likewise, all children took turns as teammates, during which time they were monitored by the team captain.

Rules for Participation General rules covering comportment and manners were developed for the class. These rules were simple and typical of many classrooms. More specific rules were developed for each of the three activities. Both sets of rules are presented in Table 2. To assist the children in recalling these rules, photos of children complying with the rules were placed in the classroom and bathroom.

Rules likewise were developed for peer-monitoring. The team captains monitored two or three classmates during the transition activities. Their rules included: 1) follow the classroom rules and set a good example; 2) remind your teammates of their duties; 3) use an inside voice, don't yell or argue; 4) give points at the end of transition; and 5) if a teammate argues, get the teacher.

Reward System Three points were available to each child each day. Each point corresponded with one of the three transition activities and could be earned by a child for completing the activity successfully. Team captains awarded the points to their teammates at the end of the three transition activities. Points were recorded under each child's name on a team chart by the monitor. Children were awarded checks individually by their monitor, in the presence of their teammates. The team charts were displayed later during a large group activity.

Rewards were based on the number of points earned. Children who earned all three checks were recognized for their performance during large group, and were eligible not only to vote for and participate in the daily recess activity but also to be appointed team captain for the next day. Children who earned two points could participate in recess but could not vote on the activity or be team captain the next day; children who earned only one point were required to remain inside for part of recess and to help clean the classroom; children who

Table 2. Class rules used in the subject alternating as client and therapist model

General Classroom Rules

1. BE A FRIEND
   Share books and games.
   Don't fight, tease, or grab.

2. BE A HELPER
   Help clean up.
   Listen to the teacher.

3. BEHAVE
   Walk, don't run.
   Sit on your mat, don't lie down.
   Be careful with classroom materials and books.

Specific Rules

1. CLEAN-UP
   Help your team to pick up.
   Ask a friend to help carry or push tables and desks—they are too heavy for one person.
   When you finish cleanup, find a mat to sit on and pick out a book.

2. BOOK TIME
   Be a friend.
   Read a book or share a book.
   Trade books when you finish one. You can go to the bookshelf two times.

3. RESTROOM
   Walk with your team.
   Use the toilet. Flush it one time.
   Wash your hands. Stay dry—don't splash.
   Wait for your team in the hall and walk back together.

4. SNACKS
   Sit on your mat.
   Wait until everyone has his or her food before you eat.
   Give your snack to the teacher if you don't want it.
   Put your leftovers and napkins in the trash when a helper brings it by.

Reprinted with permission from Carden-Smith, L., & Fowler, S. A. (1984). Positive peer pressure: The effects of peer-monitoring on children's disruptive behavior. *Journal of Applied Behavior Analysis, 17*, 213–227.

earned no points were required to remain inside for the duration of recess. Each child's reward was independent of a teammate's reward.

Training   Training was conducted prior to the introduction of the peer-monitoring intervention. Children frequently rehearsed the rules during a daily group instruction time and discussed behaviors that deserved points as well as those that did not. They also role-played point awards. Peer monitoring was introduced to the classroom once the children demonstrated through group instruction and role-plays that they knew the rules. Once peer-monitoring began, the teacher reviewed the class rules and monitoring rules immediately before the transition period with those children who were serving as team captains for the first time.

The teacher initially supervised all point awards and corrected the monitor if the point award was inaccurate. During the first three days of the peer-monitoring intervention, the teacher reminded the monitors of the procedures and of their duties. Supervision of point awards continued for several weeks. The teacher then ceased providing corrective feedback to team captains and intervened only if a dispute developed between the team captain and teammates.

Assessments   Daily observations were conducted with all children in the classroom to determine the impact of intervention on participation and disruptive behavior. Continuous interval observations were collected with the three most disruptive children in each class. A simple checklist, similar to the one used by the team captains, also was completed with all children in the class.

Figures 2 and 3 present the observational data collected with the three most disruptive children from each classroom. The figures show that the peer-monitoring procedure was successful in reducing these children's disruption and in increasing their participation. Figure 2 represents the three children from the first experiment. In this initial experiment, a teacher-monitoring condition preceded the peer monitoring condition. The second experiment, presented in Figure 3, examined whether peer monitoring could be effective without a preceding teacher condition. This experiment was conducted 1 year after the first experiment with a new class of children. The data indicate that peer-monitoring successfully reduced disruption and increased participation. The procedure continued to be effective even after teacher feedback to the monitor was withdrawn during the final condition.

Maintenance of treatment effects was not assessed in this study, due to the brevity of the summer sessions. However, the second experiment examined the effectiveness of a reduced package (peer-monitoring without teacher correction) and demonstrated that children continued to exhibit desirable rates of participation. Generalization of behavior change across settings also was not assessed in this study, as there were no other group transition times during the class day.

Consumer satisfaction surveys were not conducted in this study. However, the popularity of the peer-monitoring procedure could be inferred from the fact that children never declined the opportunity to serve as a team captain.

In summary, the results of this study suggest that children can alternate the role of therapist and client. The observational data suggest that most children behaved in a comparable fashion on days in which they were monitored and on days in which they were the monitor or team captain. Again, monitors were reluctant to withhold points from teammates and were most reluctant to withhold one of their own points. As in the subject as client model, children indicated informally that they liked the procedure by always accepting the opportunity to serve as a team captain.

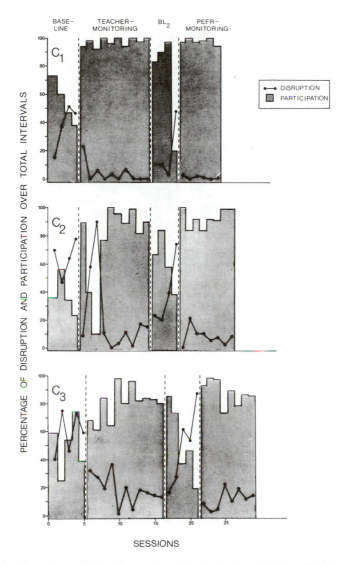

Figure 2. Percentage of disruption and participation by target children C^1, C^2, and C^3 in Experiment 1 as compared to total intervals (see discussion in text). (Reprinted with permission from Carden-Smith, L., & Fowler, S.A. [1984]. Positive peer pressure: The effects of peer-monitoring on children's disruptive behavior. *Journal of Applied Behavior Analysis, 17*, 213–227.)

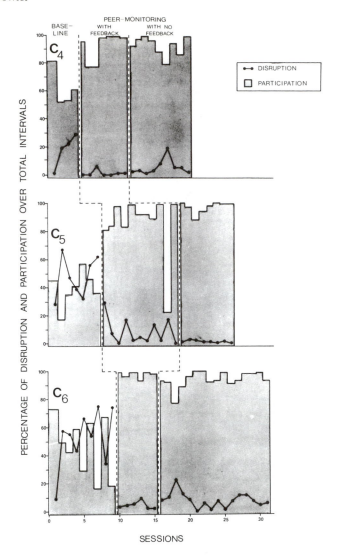

Figure 3. Percentage of disruption and participation by target children C[4], C[5], and C[6] in Experiment 2 as compared to total intervals (see discussion in text). (Reprinted with permission from Carden-Smith, L., & Fowler, S.A. [1984]. Positive peer pressure: The effects of peer-monitoring on children's disruptive behavior. *Journal of Applied Behavior Analysis*, *17*, 213–227.)

The Subject as Therapist Model

A study conducted by Fowler et al. (1986) illustrates this model. Three first-grade boys with a history of negative peer interactions were appointed to monitor individual classmates during the daily noon recess. As in the preceding Dougherty et al. (1985) study, the three peer monitors awarded points to classmates for good playing, and on rare occasions withdrew points for negative or aggressive interactions. The three boys immediately decreased their own rates of negative interactions during the sessions in which they were appointed to monitor. The following procedures were used during the study.

Criteria for Participation In this study, the three children with the highest rates of negative interactions in their class were selected to serve as peer monitors. Screening observations used for selection were conducted during the first month of school. Children's rates of positive and negative interactions were recorded during daily recess.

Six children were selected from the 19 classmates to serve as monitored peers during the first peer-monitoring condition (approximately 4 weeks in duration). Selection was based on their high sociometric ratings and appropriate play behavior. During later conditions, all members of the class, with the exception of the three subjects, took turns being monitored.

Rules for Participation Thirteen playground rules were identified and rehearsed with all members of the class prior to the collection of baseline data. The rules were posted in the classroom and were frequently reviewed during the monitoring conditions. Likewise, rules governing the monitor's behavior were introduced. The same rules were used in this study as were developed for the Dougherty et al. (1985) study.

Reward System The children who were monitored began recess with two points, which could be withdrawn one at a time following a negative interaction. In addition, the children had the opportunity to earn four bonus points for good behavior. Bonus points, once awarded, could not be withdrawn. The monitors counted the point awards and fines by using two strands of beads, which were attached to their coats or belts.

Children who met the criterion for point awards could participate in a small-group activity (concept sorting and matching games) with their monitor immediately after recess. If a child did not earn enough points, neither the child nor the monitor could participate in the activity. Points also were posted in the classroom and were accumulated for a class reward (e.g., filmstrip viewing, games), which was available at the end of the week. All members of the class participated in this activity.

Training The three boys, Adam, Bob, and Chuck, received 30 minutes of individual training, which focused on identification of appropriate and inappropriate playground behavior, opportunities for point awards, and reasons for point fines. The boys also rehearsed point award and point fine procedures. Prior to the first peer-monitoring condition, the monitoring program was described to the first-grade class, and an hour of social skills training was conducted with the class. Peer-monitoring subsequently was implemented during the noon recess. At a later time it was extended to the morning recess.

An adult was present during all recesses throughout the first peer-monitoring condition to supervise the monitors. The adult praised the monitors' performance two to three times per recess during the first appointment condition and likewise prompted them to monitor 2–10 times per recess. The adult discontinued prompts and praise to Adam and Chuck during the second appointment condition and reduced the rate of prompts and praise directed to Bob to one or two per recess. During the later phases of the study, the adult was present on the playground only intermittently.

Assessment Continuous observation data were collected with the children, who served as monitors in both intervention and nonintervention settings. In addition, consumer satisfaction data were collected with the participants of the intervention. As in the Dougherty et al. (1985) study, children appointed as monitors rated their monitoring tasks as "liked" and rated the use of point fines as "not liked." In fact, the peer monitors only withdrew a total of seven points throughout the study. Children who were monitored also rated their role as "liked." In addition, children rarely declined an opportunity to be monitored.

The direct effects of intervention on the three boys' behavior are presented in Figure 4. The appointment as peer monitor condition immediately reduced the rate of negative interaction exhibited by the three children. Each boy's negative interactions decreased from one negative interaction every 1–2 minutes to approximately one every 10 minutes. The effects were replicated with Adam and Chuck in two subsequent conditions. The effects produced with Bob in subsequent conditions were not so powerful.

Positive interactions also were affected. Bob and Chuck showed a dramatic increase in their rate of positive interactions, nearly doubling the frequency with which they interacted positively. Adam's baseline rate already was very high and did not change.

Maintenance of the effects was mixed. Once the appointment as peer monitor was withdrawn, the three boys increased their rate of negative interactions. Interestingly, Bob and Chuck maintained the high rates of positive interaction, however, that they had established during their appointment as peer monitor. Adam's positive interactions, which occurred at a high rate during the initial baseline, remained high throughout the condition changes.

Data were not collected directly with children who were monitored by the three subjects. However, the monitored peers tended to play with the monitor

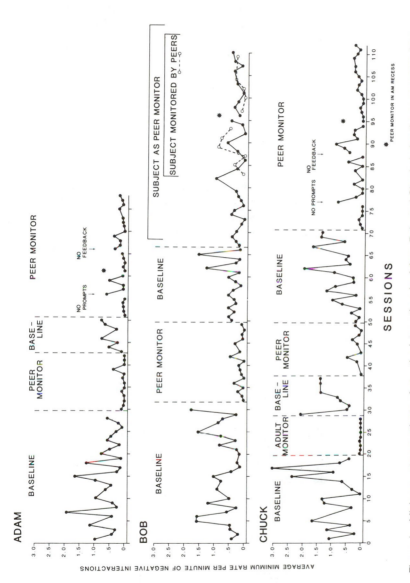

Figure 4. Minimum rate per minute of negative interactions by Adam, Bob, and Chuck during the noon recess (see discussion in text). (Reprinted with permission from Fowler, S.A., Dougherty, B.S., Kirby, K.C., & Kohler, F.W. [1986]. Role reversals: An analysis of therapeutic effects achieved with disruptive boys during their appointments as peer monitors. *Journal of Applied Behavior Analysis, 19*, 437–444.)

163

for half or more of the recess during the initial monitoring condition. During this condition, negative interactions from peers to the subject declined substantially. On the average, only one negative from a peer was directed to the monitor every 10 minutes, which contrasts with three or four negatives per 10-minute period, observed during the preceding baseline.

Two other daily recesses were observed to determine if the effects produced with the peer monitors were likely to generalize to other settings or times. Systematic decreases in negative interactions or increases in positive interactions were not evident. This result contrasts with the result obtained in the Dougherty et al. (1985) study, in which several of the monitors showed improved performance in a third setting after being appointed to monitor in two other settings.

In summary, the results of this study support the notion that appointment to the role of peer monitor can function as an intervention in itself. The three subjects reduced their rate of negative interactions during recesses in which they monitored classmates. The accuracy with which they monitored classmates was not assessed in this study. The boys typically awarded two to four bonus points to their buddy each recess and very rarely delivered a point fine. Finally, the procedure worked with very little teacher supervision during the recess period.

MAJOR ISSUES IN PEER-MEDIATED INTERVENTIONS

The three studies just presented as examples of peer-monitoring models demonstrate that children can significantly and positively influence their classmates' comportment by awarding points for appropriate behavior and withholding or withdrawing points for inappropriate behavior. The three models of peer-monitoring appear to hold promise as a potentially popular and effective set of procedures for managing behavior in group settings. Yet, a number of questions still remain regarding the practicality of the models and their potential costs and risks. These concerns, delineated next, should be addressed by educators and therapists before developing, selecting, or implementing a peer-monitoring program.

Define the Role of the Adult in Peer-Monitoring

First, the role of the adult in peer-monitoring should be delineated. To what extent is a peer-monitored intervention really managed by peers? What are the adult costs in the interventions? Peer-monitoring should not be regarded as an effective, efficient alternative to adult-monitoring until the role that adults play in mediating the peer-implemented intervention has been critically assessed. The role of the adult may vary from one intervention to another. However, adult

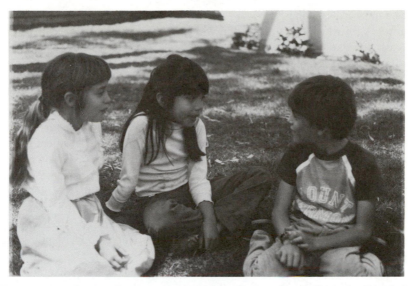

Peers can be trained to manage each other's behavior in a constructive and positive fashion. For example, arranging a group contingency can increase classmates' cooperation with or support for the monitoring procedure.

roles common to most of the interventions include: 1) training the monitors; 2) maintaining the paraphernalia associated with monitoring (e.g., the check sheets or counting beads for counting point awards and fines); 3) arranging for individual and group rewards; and 4) supervising the monitoring, at least initially.

In addition, the adult may prompt the monitor to engage in monitoring behavior or to model exemplary behavior, may praise the monitor for monitoring, and at the end of the session may provide feedback regarding the monitoring. The rate of prompts should be examined closely. If monitors act only after they are prompted by an adult, then the procedure is not very practical or efficient, and in actuality, is not a peer-monitoring procedure; rather, it is an adult-prompted monitoring procedure. The peer-monitoring procedure should be carefully supervised and assisted during the first few days following its introduction. Whenever possible, the adult's participation during the monitored activity then should be reduced across time until it is either eliminated or held at a low and constant level, as was demonstrated in the three sample studies presented in this chapter.

Assess the Accuracy or Fairness of Point Awards

The second issue that needs to be addressed in relation to a peer-monitoring program relates to the accuracy or fairness of point awards. How accurate are peers in awarding points? How accurate do they need to be? The accuracy or fairness with which peers award and withhold points has not always been assessed. Inaccurate point awards potentially risk the effectiveness of the procedure. But the risk may depend on certain circumstances. In the three studies presented in this chapter, children serving as peer monitors were very inaccurate at withholding points from peers who misbehaved. When monitors withdrew points, they typically withdrew them for very salient forms of misbehavior, such as shouting or fighting. Their failure to withdraw points contingently following less salient misbehavior did not seem to affect future rates of misbehavior, however. The monitored children's behavior either improved or was maintained at improved rates, despite the inconsistent and clearly reluctant use of point fines by the peer monitors. Finally, point fines obviously were not a popular procedure, as evidenced by monitor responses on a consumer satisfaction survey. Conversely, children were consistently generous in awarding points for good behaviors. And children consistently rated point awards as very positive.

Although point fines were not used in a malicious or vindictive fashion, the potential for their misuse exists. The current results suggest that point fines were not a crucial part of the procedure and could be deleted until demonstrated to be necessary. In fact, future research should determine the circumstances in which point awards are useful. Point awards or checks are a clear and tangible way for children to communicate to peers that they approve of their behavior; however, programs should work to eventually replace points with other social reinforcers.

Examine the Generalization and Durability of Treatment Gains

The third issue pertains to the need to evaluate the generalizability and durability of treatment gains. Are interventions mediated by peers likely to be more enduring? Are treatment changes in one child likely to produce changes in other children? Are the effects likely to extend beyond treatment settings?

A response to the first question, "Are interventions likely to be more enduring?", appears to be yes, at least sometimes. In the two recess studies (Dougherty et al., 1985; Fowler et al., 1986), subjects whose positive interactions were low prior to intervention increased those interactions and maintained those increases when treatment was withdrawn. Results were far more mixed regarding maintenance of reduced negative interactions. In the Fowler et al. (1986) study (see subject as therapist model), the three boys, Adam, Bob, and Chuck, who were appointed as monitors, did not maintain their reduced rates during reversals to baseline. In the Dougherty et al. (1985) study (see subject as client model), Dennis, who was monitored by classmates, did maintain lower rates in a follow-up study conducted 3 months after intervention. His classmates who monitored him extended their improved rates to sessions in which they were not monitoring.

Additional examples are required before we can accurately determine why treatment effects are maintained in some cases and not in others. Perhaps intermittent appointment of students as monitors may be more effective in promoting maintenance than daily appointments. The maintenance exhibited by Dennis's monitors who took turns monitoring him is striking and worth further investigation.

Are treatment effects in one child likely to produce treatment effects in other children? The answer appears to be yes, at least somewhat. In the two recess studies (Dougherty et al., 1985; Fowler et al., 1986), peers consistently decreased the frequency with which they directed negative interactions to the subjects during intervention conditions. Their reduction in negatives was closely correlated with the subjects' reductions in negatives. According to Patterson et al. (1976), children who most frequently display aggressive behaviors also are the most likely to be the victims of aggressive behavior from others. The peer-monitoring system appears to be an efficient method for breaking this cycle and for replacing negative responses with positive alternative responses. Again, these positive effects were limited to conditions in which peer-monitoring was implemented, and did not extend beyond those conditions.

It would be interesting to determine what peer responses were made to the subjects' positive interactions as well. Positive interactions typically increased during the initial peer monitoring conditions and these increases were maintained across all subsequent conditions. This author and her colleagues did not record positive actions from peers and so do not know if the subjects' increases in positive behavior were likewise met by increases in peers' responses and initiations to them. The author suspects that they may have been, however, and such results would have been consistent with the social skills literature (cf. Charlesworth & Hartup, 1967; Hendrickson et al., 1982).

Finally, are treatment effects likely to extend beyond treatment settings? The answer to this question so far is that the likelihood is not very promising. Most of the children clearly discriminated the settings in which intervention had been introduced, and did not generalize changes to other times or settings of the day. Perhaps components of the intervention program, such as the point system and assignment of peers to monitor or be monitored, exerted sufficient stimulus control to limit generalization. It would be interesting to determine if a reduced package, such as merely assigning a "buddy" in an untreated setting, would prompt at least some changes.

Risks Associated with Peer-Monitoring

Finally, potential risks associated with monitoring procedures should be addressed. What are the risks? How can they be minimized? The risk that peers will use coercion in monitoring or that peers will retaliate against monitors can be minimized through training, adult supervision of the program, and the development of a reward system that promotes cooperative behavior.

The reinforcement systems used in these studies at least initially set criterion between 50% and 75% of the available points. This criterion guaranteed that a child could receive feedback from the monitor regarding low rates of unacceptable behavior, without losing his or her reward. In some cases, bonus incentives were provided for earning all available points.

In interventions that do not involve all members of the class, a group contingency should be considered. In this procedure, the reward earned by the children who receive points is provided to all members of the class. For instance, the monitored children may exchange their points at the end of the week in order for their entire class to view a filmstrip or to take a brief field trip. Group contingencies often increase classmates' cooperation with or support for the monitoring procedure.

Careful training was provided prior to the introduction of each monitoring procedure. Training in the form of role-plays and rehearsals was provided to the children participating directly in the monitoring procedure. The monitors also received training to provide positive feedback to peers. During the initial days of the intervention, the adult either introduced the procedure (as in a brief adult-monitoring condition) or provided close supervision to the monitors. Feedback was also provided at the end of the session regarding the quality of monitoring. Finally, in two of the studies, satisfaction and discomfort resulting from peer-monitoring were routinely assessed with both the monitored children and the monitors. Likewise, accuracy of point awards was assessed.

SUMMARY

In summary, children are an extremely useful resource to each other and to the adults who are responsible for their supervision. The three models of peer monitoring presented in this chapter demonstrate ways in which children can be trained to manage one another's behavior problems constructively and positively. The three monitoring procedures provide a framework for children to maintain behavior changes, initially established by adults. They also provide, in at least some cases, sufficiently powerful procedures for children to establish the initial behavior change. Just as important, each procedure provides peers with a set of behaviors that supports the behavior changes of the child receiving the intervention, whether the peer assumes the role of therapist or client. Additional research is still required to determine ways in which peers can support and extend behavior change consistently beyond the intervention time and setting.

REFERENCES

Carden-Smith, L., & Fowler, S.A. (1984). Positive peer pressure: The effects of peer monitoring on children's disruptive behavior. *Journal of Applied Behavior Analysis, 17*, 213–227.

Charlesworth, R., & Hartup, W.W. (1967). Positive social reinforcement in the nursery school peer group. *Child Development, 38*, 993–1002.

Dougherty, B.S., Fowler, S.A., & Paine, S. (1985). The use of peer monitors to reduce negative interactions during recess. *Journal of Applied Behavior Analysis, 18*, 141–153.

Drabman, R.S. (1973). Child versus teacher-administered token programs in a psychiatric hospital school. *Journal of Abnormal Child Psychology, 1*, 68–87.

Egel, A.L., Richman, G.S., & Koegel, R.L. (1981). Normal peer models and autistic children's learning. *Journal of Applied Behavior Analysis, 14*, 3–12.

Fowler, S.A. (1986). Peer-monitoring and self-monitoring: Alternatives to traditional teacher management. *Exceptional Children, 52*, 573–581.

Fowler, S.A., Dougherty, B.S., Kirby, K.C., & Kohler, F.W. (1986). Role reversals: An analysis of therapeutic effects achieved with disruptive boys during their appointments as peer monitors. *Journal of Applied Behavior Analysis, 19*, 437–444.

Goldstein, H., & Wickstrom, S. (1986). Programming maintenance after correspondence training interventions with children. *Journal of Applied Behavior Analysis, 19*, 209–214.

Greenwood, C.R., & Hops, H. (1981). Group-oriented contingencies and peer behavior change. In P.S. Strain (Ed.), *The utilization of classroom peers as behavior change agents* (pp. 189–259). New York: Plenum.

Greenwood, C.R., Sloane, H.N., Jr., & Baskin, A. (1974). Training elementary aged peer behavior managers to control small group programmed mathematics. *Journal of Applied Behavior Analysis, 7*, 103–114.

Hendrickson, J.M., Strain, P.S., Tremblay, A., & Shores, R.E. (1982). Interactions of behaviorally handicapped children: Functional effects of peer social initiations. *Behavior Modification, 6*, 323–353.

Johnston, J.M., & Johnston, G.T. (1972). Modification of consonant speech-sound articulation in young children. *Journal of Applied Behavioral Analysis, 5*, 233–246.

Kazdin, A.E. (1977). *The token economy: A review and evaluation.* New York: Plenum.

Kohler, F.W., & Fowler, S.A. (1985). Training prosocial behaviors to young children: An analysis of reciprocity with untrained peers. *Journal of Applied Behavior Analysis, 18*, 187–200.

Lancioni, G.E. (1982). Normal children as tutors to teach social responses to withdrawn mentally retarded schoolmates: Training, maintenance, and generalization. *Journal of Applied Behavior Analysis, 15*, 17–40.

Odom, S.L., & Strain, P.S. (1986). A comparison of peer-initiation and teacher-antecedent interventions for promoting reciprocal social interaction of autistic preschoolers. *Journal of Applied Behavior Analysis, 19*, 59–71.

Patterson, G.R., Littman, R.A., & Bricker, W. (1976). Assertive behavior in children: A step toward a theory of aggression. *Monographs of the Society for Research in Child Development, 32* (Serial No. 113).

Phillips, E.L., Phillips, E.A., Wolf, M.M., & Fixsen, D.L. (1973). Achievement place: Development of the elected manager system. *Journal of Applied Behavior Analysis, 6*, 541–561.

Sainato, D.M., Maheady, L., & Shook, G.L. (1986). The effects of a classroom manager role on the social interaction patterns and social status of withdrawn kindergarten students. *Journal of Applied Behavior Analysis, 19,* 187–195.

Schreibman, L., O'Neill, R.E., & Koegel, R.L. (1983). Behavioral training for siblings of autistic children. *Journal of Applied Behavior Analysis, 16,* 129–138.

Shafer, M.S., Egel, A.L., & Neef, N.A. (1984). Training mildly handicapped peers to facilitate changes in the social interaction skills of autistic children. *Journal of Applied Behavior Analysis, 17,* 461–476.

Solomon, R.W., & Wahler, R.G. (1973). Peer reinforcement control of classroom problem behavior. *Journal of Applied Behavior Analysis, 6,* 49–56.

Stokes, T.F., & Baer, D.M. (1976). Preschool peers as mutual generalization-facilitation agents. *Behavior Therapy, 7,* 549–556.

Strain, P.S. (1983). Identification of social skill curriculum targets for severely handicapped children in mainstreamed preschools. *Applied Research in Mental Retardation, 4,* 369–382.

Strain, P.S., Kerr, M.M., & Ragland, E.U. (1981). The use of peer social initiations in the treatment of social withdrawal. In P.S. Strain (Ed.), *The utilization of classroom peers as behavior change agents* (pp. 101–128). New York: Plenum.

Twardosz, S., Nordquist, V.M., Simon, R., Botkin, D. (1983). The effect of group affection activities on the interaction of socially isolate children. *Analysis and Intervention in Developmental Disabilities, 3,* 311–338.

Walker, H.M., Hops, H., Greenwood, C.R., Todd, N.M., Street, A., & Garrett, B. (1978). *The comparative effects of teacher praise, token reinforcement, and response cost in reducing negative peer interactions (Report No. 25).* Eugene: University of Oregon, Center at Oregon for Research in the Behavioral Education of the Handicapped.

Warren, S.F., Baer, D.M., & Rogers-Warren, A. (1979). Teaching children to praise: A problem in stimulus and response generalization. *Child Behavior Therapy, 1,* 160–175.

Chapter 8

Generalizing and Maintaining Improvement in Problem Behavior

Judith E. Favell and Dennis H. Reid

Over the last 25 years there has been a concerted and continuing effort to develop, refine, and extend methods of treating problem behavior among individuals with developmental disabilities. Literally hundreds of studies have provided convincing evidence that problems such as aggression, self-injury, property damage, and other destructive and disruptive behavior can be systematically decreased (Judith Favell, McGimsey, & Schell, 1982; Whitman, Scibak, & Reid, 1983). Effective treatment strategies have included individual and composite variations of rearranging antecedent events, differential reinforcement of appropriate alternative behavior, and arranging consequences for the problem itself (*Journal of Applied Behavior Analysis,* 1968–1985).

While the technology of treatment continues to evolve, researchers and practitioners are also attempting to address the limitations of that technology. Among these limitations, perhaps the most challenging relates to our ability to effect pervasive, durable improvement in problem behavior. Although it may be possible to suppress a problem in a circumscribed, controlled situation, practitioners often fail to change behavior in all clinically relevant situations. For example, although a client's aggression may be successfully treated in school, it may nevertheless continue to occur at the same or higher level at

---

Dr. Favell is currently with the Au Clair Program, Carlton Palms Education Center, Mount Dora, Florida 32757.

home. Further, although treatment may be effective initially, durable improvement may not result and, instead, the problem gradually (or even precipitiously) returns as weeks or months elapse. In short, despite indisputable evidence that the technology of behavior analysis can produce clinically significant results with problem behavior, these claims must be carefully qualified with common limitations in the generalization and maintenance of these gains.

The research literature provides limited help in substantiating the extent of the problem with generalization and maintenance, in identifying possible explanations, or in addressing potential solutions. Most studies treat generalization and maintenance on a very limited scale. Typically treatment is applied for relatively short durations (e.g., 30-minute sessions), and generalization, if assessed at all, is measured or programmed in a small number of "extra therapy" time periods or settings. Similarly, maintenance of improvement is commonly tracked only across weeks or possibly a few months following treatment. Occasionally, follow-up data from individual observations conducted at spaced intervals are also included. Thus, the empirical literature continues to reflect a relatively narrow focus despite the recognition that clinically significant effects are truly achieved only when severe problems are brought under control in all life situations and when these improvements are maintained for years.

The relative dearth of research may reflect several realities associated with addressing the issue of generalization and maintenance. First, work in this area is, by definition, extremely labor-intensive, requiring extensive resources to measure and program behavior change across extended periods of time. Second, even when clinical researchers can garner the necessary resources to conduct such research, the professional rewards can be lean. Professionals, often under pressure to publish, may avoid single studies that require months and years to complete. But perhaps most important, research on generalization and maintenance confronts researchers with a myriad of factors over which they often have little control. Although it may be relatively easy to work with clients in a circumscribed setting, measuring and programming for generalization and maintenance outside that controlled setting is quite another matter. Reliable measurement systems must be established to accurately detect occurrences of the problem behavior, caregivers must be taught to apply the treatment procedures in all clinically relevant situations, and steps must be taken to ensure that the treatment is conducted correctly and consistently. The difficulties and complexities of this process cannot be overstated when researchers have little functional authority over the program and staff, and in service systems that often operate with too few resources and too many clients with challenging needs.

What literature does exist does not provide particularly encouraging accounts of the durability of improvement. In three major follow-up studies of retarded and autistic clients with behavior problems, results revealed regression—for example, the loss of skills and return of problems in many instances (Foxx & Livesay, 1984; Lovaas, Koegel, Simmons, & Long, 1973; Schroeder et al., 1982). Similar accounts of circumscribed and temporary effects are unfortunately common in the clinical trenches. However, the lack of research and the guarded outlook described in the available literature do not have to imply that the field must settle for limited clinical outcomes. There are a variety of trends and factors that hold promise in both improving the effectiveness of initial treatment and in enhancing the likelihood of successful generalization and maintenance.

DESIGNING TREATMENT

Over the years, changes have occurred in the way treatment is conceptualized, designed, and applied. These changes offer hope not only for improving the effectiveness of initial treatment but also for contributing to successful generalization and maintenance as well.

Treatment Based on the Functional Analysis of Problem Behavior

In recent years, increasing attention has been paid to examining problem behavior in its ecological context, attempting to detect how it varies across conditions and what contingencies may be maintaining it. One of the earliest and most important discoveries in the field of behavior analysis was that problem behavior such as self-injury serves a function for the individual, that it is maintained by its consequences (Lovaas, Freitag, Gold, & Kassorla, 1965). From that general premise, research since the mid-1970s has provided more precise details of specific mechanisms of reinforcement for problem behavior (Carr, 1977). It is now clear that positive reinforcement such as attention (Lovaas & Simmons, 1969), negative reinforcement such as escape from demands (Carr, Newsom, & Binkoff, 1980), and possibly sensory reinforcement (Judith Favell, McGimsey, & Schell, 1982; Rincover, Cook, Peoples, & Packard, 1979) can maintain problem behavior.

Increased interest and information in motivational mechanisms have led to the development of methods of analyzing the function of problems in individual cases. These methods are designed to examine behavior in the context of various environmental events, in an attempt to identify conditions and contingencies maintaining the problem. Several specific methods of conducting ecological or functional analysis have been described (Iwata, Dorsey, Slifer, Bauman, & Richman, 1982; LaVigna & Donnellan, 1986; Touchette, MacDonald, & Langer, 1985).

Some methods involve a laboratory analogue procedure in which clients are exposed to different antecedent and consequent events under controlled conditions (Iwata et al., 1982). When a client self-injures differentially under conditions in which high demands are presented, for example, and the behavior is consequated by termination of those demands, but self-injures less in low-demand situations, it is concluded that the behavior is serving an escape function (i.e., it is negatively reinforced). When self-injury occurs instead in the presence of people who attend to it, but not when the client is alone and ignored, a positive reinforcement paradigm is inferred.

A second type of approach to a functional or ecological analysis was conducted by Touchette et al. (1985), who tracked clients across naturalistic conditions and recorded their behavior using a scatter plot grid. At times in which the behavior occurred frequently or intensely, the corresponding grid was fully darkened. At times when the problem occurred at a low frequency or not at all, the grid was half-filled or not marked, respectively. In this way a profile of darkly shaded areas reveals times, places, activities, and people that are differentially associated with the problem. Such a profile enables a more detailed scrutiny of each high probability situation, from which information on specific conditions and contingencies maintaining the problem may be derived.

Regardless of the specific method employed, the importance and potential benefits of conducting ecological or functional analyses are becoming clear. Such analyses offer assurance of increasing our general understanding of the development and maintenance of problem behavior, enabling the accumulation of increasingly precise information about how common antecedent and consequent events function to shape and maintain these problems.

Aside from its heuristic value, it is hoped that functional analysis will have immediate clinical utility by improving our prescriptive power (i.e., by increasing the effectiveness of our initial treatment and by enhancing the generality and maintenance of those effects). Research is needed to explore whether functional analysis actually results in improved clinical outcomes relative to prescriptions devised in the absence of such information. Nevertheless, the logic and face validity seem promising. Treatment based on information about how varying situations differentially control the problem and probable functions the behavior serves may enhance treatment effectiveness by altering the functional properties of clients' environments, correcting conditions and contingencies maintaining the problem, and rearranging natural events to better support more appropriate behavior. Without functional impact on conditions and contingencies maintaining a problem, limited effects in treatment and especially in generalization and maintenance can be expected. Too often, sound and potentially effective treatment is superimposed on ongoing environments that continue to inadvertently maintain the problem. In these instances, treatment competes with and often loses against these naturally occurring conditions, resulting in negligible treatment effects or the gradual erosion of even promising initial results. Such common results are often said to be due to weak treatment technology. That may be true in a relative sense, that is, treatment techniques may be weak *relative* to the operation of powerful ambient variables that continue unchecked, competing for behavioral control during treatment periods and especially having an impact on behavior when treatment is diluted, as in generalization and maintenance phases. Thus, prescriptions derived from functional or ecological analyses may prove superior to treatment programs that are more arbitrarily conceived, because the former may set the occasion for rearranging and correcting natural variables that are sustaining problem behavior—variables that if not addressed, are likely to compete with initial treatment effectiveness and certainly with generalization and maintenance efforts.

Treatment Based on Developing Functional Alternatives

In recent years, increasing emphasis has been placed on treating problems by teaching and reinforcing appropriate alternative behavior. In early work, such an approach was sometimes absent altogether or given only an academic nod in interventions that principally concentrated on using consequences for inappropriate behavior. The latter orientation is steadily being reversed in research and practice.

The essential notion is that as appropriate behavior is differentially reinforced relative to problem behavior, rates of the latter should decline. In the

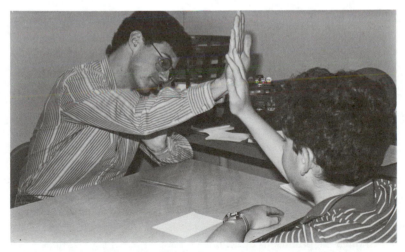

Reinforcing appropriate alternative behaviors to decrease problem behaviors.

most basic application of this approach, "differential reinforcement of other behavior" (DRO), reinforcement is presented following intervals in which the problem behavior has not occurred and is delayed when it does occur (Dietz & Repp, 1983). A more focused version of differential reinforcement involves targeting appropriate behavior that it is hoped will prove to be "functionally incompatible" with the problem. Functionally incompatible responses are those that vary in the opposite direction when intervention is applied to one response. Thus, if face slapping is not directly treated, but decreases systematically when appropriate use of leisure materials is increased with reinforcement, then these behaviors are termed functionally incompatible. The literature contains a variety of demonstrations of treating behavior problems by targeting appropriate behavior that is functionally incompatible with it. For example, in a recent and well-controlled study, Parrish, Cataldo, Kolko, Neef, and Egel (1986) demonstrated that compliance in young children covaried inversely with a variety of inappropriate behaviors. If, for example, instruction-following was reinforced, aggression and disruption systematically declined without direct intervention.

Much research remains to be done to identify what and why behaviors become functionally incompatible. However, treatments based on covariation hold great promise as efficient and benign behavior-change strategies. Not only can multiple outcomes be achieved with intervention on a single behavior, but when the intervention involves reinforcing appropriate behavior, problems may be treated with no suppressive consequence (see Horner and Billingsly, Chapter 9).

As explorations of functional incompatibility continue, another concept, that of "functional equivalence," has emerged. This concept is based on the premise that treatment of behavior problems may be enhanced by not only reinforcing alternative and incompatible behavior but, more precisely, by targeting behavior that will achieve the same *function* that previously only the problem behavior achieved. The operations necessary for such an approach involve identifying the reinforcers maintaining the problem behavior and arranging for other, appropriate responses to produce the same or similar reinforcers. Functional equivalents, then, are behaviors that differ in form but serve the same function. The hope is that teaching functional equivalents will result in more effective treatments, for example, because they inherently reduce the necessity or motivation for engaging in the behavior problem. Perhaps most importantly, it is hoped that such a strategy will enhance generalization and maintenance of improvement by providing clients with new skills that can be used in all settings and at all times that the problem was used previously to achieve similar purposes (cf. Carr, Chapter 10).

Although the promise is clear, much research remains to be done to confirm and elaborate these possibilities. In a pioneering example, Carr and Durand (1985) demonstrated that various problems such as tantrums and self-injury by autistic students occurred under low levels of adult attention and high levels of task difficulty. Teaching these children communication skills to recruit attention and/or assistance from adults systematically and decisively decreased these problems. Through research such as this, it is expected that the therapeutic benefits of teaching functional equivalents will be elaborated.

The efficacy of functional equivalence may ultimately rest on whether the alternative behavior is as effective, efficient, and reliable in obtaining reinforcement as the problem that it is intended to replace. The dimension of "effectiveness" surrounds the issue of what type of reinforcer is produced by the appropriate behavior. As just indicated, the concept of functional equivalence rests on the assumption that the form of reinforcement for appropriate behavior must be the same or similar to that which follows the problem behavior. However, it is possible that equivalence in *potency* is as or more essential to effective treatment than matches in form. Thus, it may be possible to employ conventional reinforcers (e.g., praise and edibles) to increase appropriate behavior, so long as these are as potent as the reinforcers maintaining the problem. The use of "arbitrary" reinforcers can have real advantages over the identification and use of reinforcers for problem behavior, which can be difficult to identify and may be considered inappropriate (e.g., disruptive or stigmatizing).

On the other hand, matches in potency may not be sufficient, particularly in generalizing and maintaining improvement. By identifying reinforcers for the problem and reconfiguring these so that they become available for less aberrant responding, the *relative* level of reinforcement is *functionally* shifted from problem behavior to appropriate responding. In contrast, even massive increases in "arbitrary" reinforcers for appropriate behavior do not necessarily alter the relative reinforcement for the problem. Though it is typically impossible to discontinue reinforcers for the problem altogether, nevertheless the relative reinforcement for the problem can be reduced through providing the individual with copious alternative means of obtaining similar reinforcers. Such a process epitomizes the basic premise that treatment of problem behavior is best approached by correcting conditions maintaining the problem and rearranging natural conditions and contingencies so as to support more appropriate behavior. Although temporary improvement may be obtained with more artificial and contrived reinforcers, the continued existence and operation of reinforcers for inappropriate behavior is likely to eventually regain dominance, especially as the more contrived reinforcers for appropriate behavior are "thinned" and otherwise altered in generalization and maintenance phases.

Demonstrations of functional incompatibility in which reinforcement of appropriate behavior results in reductions in aberrant behavior may rest not only on the effectiveness of the appropriate behavior in producing reinforcement but also on the relative "efficiency" and "reliability" with which the appropriate behavior achieves those ends. Two responses may produce the same reinforcer, but one may nevertheless have many more opportunities to occur, may require less effort or otherwise be easier to display—that is, it may be more efficient than the other (cf. Horner and Billingsley, Chapter 9). Similarly, one response may produce reinforcement more reliably (i.e., at a higher ratio) than the other. For example, although two behaviors may each be effective in gaining a break from work in class, raising one's hand may be unobtrusive, time-consuming, and subject to conditional reinforcement rules (may only be reinforced at certain times). On the other hand, throwing a book at another student suffers from none of these drawbacks and is likely to produce a break from routine much more efficiently and reliably.

The fact that more efficient and reliable responses may dominate over less efficient and reliable behaviors may account for reduced effectiveness in initial treatment efforts with reinforcement procedures, and in poor generalization and maintenance of effects. A common set of problems in communication training may serve as an example. First, the communicative responses targeted may be appropriate but not effective in gaining reinforcement similar to that which the problem produced. In an obvious example, although teaching a student to sign "juice" may be desirable, that response may have no relevance to her outbursts of aggression, which may function chiefly to drive peers away. Second, the selection of communicative skills must be based in part on the ease with which clients can learn and display them. If weeks of training in a difficult signing response are necessary, the client is likely to resort to easier, though inappropriate, forms of communication. Finally, the communication skill must be recognized and reinforced by all on a reliable basis. Given this need, the focus of training shifts from the client to caregivers in his or her social environment, teaching and ensuring that communicative attempts are reinforced more reliably (i.e., at a higher ratio) than their inappropriate counterparts. The need to ensure that reinforcement is reliable cannot be overstated. The current emphasis on training alternative behavior must be matched with the recognition that such efforts often fail, not during the initial stages, but beyond intensive training. Although training alternative appropriate behavior is not easy, it is often easier than ensuring that skills, once acquired, continue to produce reinforcement reliability.

In general, when behaviors selected for training are appropriate but not effective in producing reinforcers that the problem behavior can produce, when these skills are difficult and time-consuming to learn and conditions are not arranged in the ambient environment so that the client is encouraged and reliably reinforced for practicing the skill, behavior problems are likely to continue unabated. In these cases, one might conclude that reinforcement for alternative behavior has failed. To the contrary, despite all good intentions, the individual has not been provided with functional alternatives that were effective, efficient, and reliable means of obtaining reinforcement, especially reinforcement that the problem behavior previously produced.

Treatment as a Comprehensive, Composite Approach

Historically, treatment was often described as consisting of an individual procedure such as differential reinforcement, overcorrection, timeout, or food satiation. Such a focus on singular and relatively narrow interventions undoubtedly reflects the appropriate scientific mandate of attempting to isolate the effects of individual treatments or elements of treatment. Although ferreting out the critical, functional components of intervention has unarguable benefit for understanding and replicating treatment, it can be clinically misleading. Regardless of the singular label applied to an intervention, treatment in fact usually consists of a myriad of changes in the client's social and physical environment. Although these alterations may be cumbersome or appear too trivial to describe in the typical journal article, they nevertheless may have figured centrally in the treatment's success. Unfortunately, the narrow, simplified descriptions appearing in the professional journals perpetrate the view that these dimensions are sufficient to ameliorate problems. In contrast, this view runs contrary to not only actual but good clinical practice. In a report describing the "state of the art" in treating self-injurious behavior, a task force convened by the Association for Advancement of Behavior Therapy (AABT) recommended that *each* intervention explicitly include *all* of the following dimensions:

> The identification of biological and environmental conditions which may maintain the client's self-injury and the explicit inclusion of that information in the design of treatment. Such an analysis should include identification of medical conditions which may contribute to the problem, environmental situations which regularly evoke the behavior, and the consequences of self-injury which may be reinforcing it.
>
> The deliberate teaching and reinforcement of noninjurious, appropriate behavior. Such behavioral alternatives to self-injury may include communication, cooperation with tasks, independent leisure, and social skills.
>
> The identification and discontinuation of reinforcers for the self-injurious behavior, typically by arranging conditions so that caretakers can safely and consistently minimize reactions to the behavior which might be inadvertently reinforcing it.
>
> The establishment and provision of overall stimulus conditions which are associated with noninjurious behavior (such as through environmental enrichment), and the alteration or elimination of environmental conditions which are regularly associated with self-injury (such as situations which are unnecessarily frustrating or nonreinforcing).

In cases where the behavior is dangerous, interferes excessively with habilitative or humanizing activities, or has failed to improve when treated with the less intrusive procedures outlined above, a punishing consequence such as overcorrection, or in extremely severe cases, shock for self-injury may also be necessary.

The provision for generalizing improvement into all environments in which the individual lives and for maintaining improvement over time. (Judith Favell, Azrin, et al., 1982)

Thus, this AABT task force recommended a composite approach, combining a variety of individual procedures, each of which addresses a different and necessary aspect of intervention. The emphasis on composite approaches reflects an increased understanding that individual elements affect only one part of the clinical picture (i.e., only one aspect of the problem). When applied in isolation, that aspect is likely to have only partial, fragmented, and delimited effects.

ARRANGING CONSEQUENCES FOR PROBLEM BEHAVIOR

One of the most significant recent shifts in the approach to treating problem behavior relates to the philosophy and practice of arranging consequences for problems. In the past and in some cases continuing into the present, treatment efforts have been criticized for concentrating on the use of "aversive" or "restrictive" consequences. Although procedures such as enforced timeout, overcorrection, and contingent use of noxious events have been demonstrated to have decisive effects in suppressing behavior problems, preoccupation with their use is associated with several problems.

Humanitarian concerns are clearly raised in cases in which restrictive consequences have been employed without prior or concurrent use of reinforcement procedures. Further, the use of punishment and timeout enabled the suppression of problem behavior without attending to the environmental conditions and contingencies maintaining the problem. Without restructuring those factors, behavioral improvement was often circumscribed and temporary, as those variables continued to provoke and reinforce the problem. These and other problems were the result of excessive or even exclusive use of "restrictive" consequences, which infringed on rights and resulted in limited clinical outcomes.

However, as movement occurs in the direction of alternative treatment strategies and away from heavy emphasis on "restrictive" consequences, it remains important to critically analyze several issues surrounding the use of punishment and timeout that bear on our ability to treat problems, and particularly that relate to issues of generalization and maintenance. First, as indicated, the use of punishment and timeout are often held *responsible* for the poor generalization and maintenance seen in many treatment efforts. A common complaint is that these procedures produce very circumscribed effects (i.e., when a behavior is punished in one situation, such as in class, but not in another, such as at home, it is likely that the problem will be reduced only in the former setting). In situations in which punishment is not employed or available, the problem will continue or even worsen (Azrin & Holz, 1966). This observation is accurate, but must be placed in its proper context, for it also applies to virtually all treatment techniques. Reinforcement for appropriate behavior has similarly circumscribed effects; if employed in one situation and not in another, it is very likely that improvement will be seen only in the situation in which reinforcement is available. The point has been made repeatedly that generalization does not typically occur naturally with *any* type of intervention (Baer, 1981; Stokes & Baer, 1977). At the present level of technology, the most reliable way of ensuring comprehensive improvement is to employ treatment in all situations. It is necessary with punishment; it is also necessary with reinforcement-based interventions. Although there may be differences in the extent of discriminability between different techniques—for example, clients form exceedingly fine discriminations with powerful punishers such as contingent shock (Birnbrauer, 1968)—this should not obscure the fact that these differences appear to be ones of degree and not of kind.

A similar point applies to the temporary effects ascribed to the use of punishment and timeout. Though it is clear that a behavior problem may return when its consequences are discontinued, this observation applies equally to all interventions. When reinforcement for appropriate behavior is no longer forthcoming, those skills are likely to deteriorate (Kazdin & Esveldt-Dawson, 1981). In short, regardless of the techniques employed, maintenance does not occur naturally, but must be planned with care and conducted with vigilance.

Criticism of poor generalization and maintenance with punishment and timeout not only overlooks similar problems with other treatment strategies but also reflects a misunderstanding of their role. The use of suppressive consequences is not intended to permanently "cure" a problem, but to initially decrease the rate of the behavior so that teaching of alternative skills can be introduced into the periods between occurrences of the misbehavior. Such teaching is difficult if not impossible when an individual is engaged in highly frequent attempts at misbehavior and when the behavior is extremely dangerous and disruptive. Thus punishment is neither intended nor justified as the sole and long-term "solution," but only as a means of reducing rates of problems to the point that teaching alternative skills is possible (Lovaas & Favell, in press).

In general, problems with generalization and maintenance associated with the use of timeout and punishment should not obscure the fact that similar problems exist with all interventions. Regardless of the strategy employed, clinicians must explicitly program for improvement across settings and over time if successful generalization and maintenance are to occur. Further, the proper role of suppressive consequences is to create "daylight" between bouts of misbehavior to enable the use of teaching procedures that will train the adaptive skills crucial in ensuring generalized and maintained improvement in behavior problems.

A second issue associated with the use of punishment and timeout bears directly on generalizing and maintaining improvement in behavior problems. Because treatment typically must be applied in all settings and continued over time, it is important that the intervention selected be acceptable and applicable in all settings in which the client functions and will function. It is common to hear that restrictive procedures are not available for use because a program, facility, or agency is not able or willing to use them. In some cases, the availability of only benign techniques does not create difficulty; the client's problem may be ameliorated with an intervention that is both effective and acceptable in all settings. However, when this is not the case, the clinician is confronted with a dilemma: to bring the problem under control with a technique that will not be available in another setting, or to use procedures that are acceptable to all but that may not be fully effective. Either alternative can functionally prohibit a client's movement to another setting. On the one hand, the procedures used to bring and keep a behavior under control are not acceptable, and on the other hand, continued occurrences of a problem may make the client ineligible for placement. Thus, the issue of what type of punishment or timeout procedures are to be employed bears directly on generalization and maintenance of improvement, for all current and future settings must be equipped and willing to employ similar interventions.

Restrictive procedures are often prohibited for two reasons. First, an agency or program may feel that it cannot ensure that the procedures are used properly and safely. This is a most legitimate concern, for these techniques can be abused or misused, with extremely deleterious effects. However, if a program does not have the resources and expertise to ensure the safe and proper use of restrictive techniques, one must ask whether that program can treat severe behavior problems at all. Restrictive procedures do not require resources and expertise; treatment of behavior problems does. In reality, punishment and timeout techniques are relatively simple to employ when compared with the subtleties and complexities associated with the proper use of differential reinforcement. Thus, proper treatment necessitates similar levels of expertise regardless of which techniques are employed. Further, one should not necessarily assume that clients are safer from abuse because restrictive procedures have been disallowed. Risks associated with a procedure must always be referenced against risks associated with lack of treatment. If a behavior problem is dangerous, lack of effective treatment places the client or his or her victims in severe jeopardy.

Given the needs and risks associated with treating severe behavior problems, the answer to safe and proper treatment does not rest with disallowing one set of restrictive techniques, but instead should be based on guaranteeing that resources and expertise are available regardless of the interventions employed. In short, the same dimensions necessary for restrictive procedures are necessary to employ any treatment safely and proficiently. If the highest standards of all dimensions of treatment cannot be guaranteed (e.g., staff training, professional expertise, administrative support, due process, and monitoring), then a program should not purport or attempt to treat severe behavior disorders by any means.

A second reason against the use of restrictive procedures in various settings in which improvement must generalize and maintain surrounds the issue of normalization. It is sometimes felt that procedures such as locked timeout or contingent restraint do not belong in certain programs (particularly in the community), and that only the most benign, natural, and normalized techniques should be employed there. It is clear that in some cases behavior problems are effectively and durably treated solely with benign and normalized means. However, in other cases an individual's behavior may not respond or may begin to deteriorate without the use of restrictive interventions. Under such conditions, too often the client is prevented from moving into a setting that does not employ the restrictive intervention or is returned to a setting that does. The practice of extruding clients whose behavior requires more intrusive, less normalized interventions is a double-edged sword. On the one hand, programs should honestly recognize what types of problems and interventions they are willing and equipped to handle. On the other hand, by returning an individual to a setting that is able/willing to use timeout or punishment but that does not meet the individual's needs in other respects, a program that extrudes an individual must bear some degree of responsibility for denying that individual the right to live in a less restrictive environment.

A third issue bearing on the use of restrictive consequences and the generalization and maintenance of improvement relates to the model of least restrictiveness. This model states that a problem should be treated with the least intrusive/restrictive methods effective in ameliorating it. The model of least restrictiveness has properly challenged clinicians to consider and attempt more benign interventions before resorting to ones that are associated with greater degrees of restrictiveness (e.g., with loss of freedom, aversiveness, susceptibility to abuse, and departure from normative practice). The humanitarian intent of such a stricture is clear and extremely important. The clinical promise, particularly in terms of generalization and maintenance, is important as well, for it may be that the more benign and natural the intervention, the greater the likelihood that it can and will be used across settings and time.

Despite the important and admirable message contained in the model of least restrictiveness, the emphasis on benign, natural, and normalized procedures has in some cases eclipsed attention to the need for *effective* interventions. In these instances, programs may select and employ procedures principally on their benign appearance, even in cases in which the procedure has no discernible effect on behavior. The unintended result is that clients are exposed to periods of ineffective procedures, with their problems continuing untreated and possibly becoming desensitized to all but the most intense intervention.

Selecting treatment on benign appearance rather than clinical efficacy has a direct bearing on the effectiveness of initial treatment efforts and on generalization and maintenance efforts as well. In some cases, problems in generalization and maintenance actually reflect poor treatment effects in the first place— that is, the behavior was not fully suppressed during treatment, and continued rates at other times are simply extensions of those original levels. Further, regardless of initial results, the effects of any treatment may be diminished as the treatment is employed by a variety of caregivers, under widely varying conditions, and continued for long periods. Although these natural variations may dilute even interventions that have extremely potent initial effects, the consequences of this possible "ripple effect" are probably more serious with interventions that produce only partial or mixed effects, when applied in their most optimal fashion. Thus, in the interest of effective initial treatment and to increase the likelihood of generalized and maintained improvement with the use of that treatment in all settings and over time, care must be taken to ensure that techniques are selected on the basis of their *effectiveness* as well as their benign appearance.

Competent and ethical therapists must be given the latitude to employ procedures that are as nonrestrictive as possible but that are also effective in reducing the problem in clinically significant ways. Given appropriate latitude in selecting techniques, therapists can then be held accountable for the treatment decisions they make. If a therapist treats problems exclusively with the use of restrictive procedures, then he or she should not be allowed to practice behavior therapy. If, on the other hand, a therapist employs only techniques that are benign in appearance but that do not effectively ameliorate problems, then he or she should similarly not be allowed to prescribe treatment.

In short, individuals and programs must be expected to select and employ interventions that are as benign as possible, but that are effective in decisively reducing problem behavior. Unless program developers and practitioners have access to a full array of procedures and the latitude to select among these treatments on the basis of their effectiveness, outcomes may remain limited.

PLANNING AND PROGRAMMING FOR GENERALIZATION AND MAINTENANCE

The definitions of *generalization* and *maintenance* point implicitly and explicitly to improvement that occurs under conditions of reduced or discontinued treatment (Kazdin & Esveldt-Dawson, 1981). Although on occasion, generalization and maintenance of improvement in behavior problems seem to occur "naturally" beyond treatment (e.g., Eason, White, & Newsom, 1982), more often they do not. Instead, the classic premise, stated years ago, is regularly reaffirmed in research and clinical practice: The effects of contingencies barely outlive their presence (Baer & Wolf, 1970). Although interventions may be developed that inherently facilitate generalization and maintenance, at the present level of technology it seems clear that the only certain way of achieving such outcomes is to program for them.

Several steps taken during initial treatment are pivotal in producing generalized and durable behavior change, particularly by avoiding practices that inadvertently limit the range of clinical outcomes. Certainly treatment should be conducted under conditions that closely resemble those existing in the client's natural environment (cf. Sailor, Goetz, Anderson, Hunt, & Gee, Chapter 4). This truism not only facilitates transfer of behavioral gains but avoids two threats to generalization and maintenance. First, it allows treatment to be developed in, and adjusted to, the realities of the individual's living environment. Treatment developed outside of the natural context too often ignores such crucial variables as the ratio and preferences of caregivers, for example, which have a direct impact upon whether treatment is possible or will be used. Many treatment efforts are doomed to failure at the outset because they contain nonreplicable elements. Factors ranging from caregiver size to voice-tone can prove pivotal, and can be detected and addressed as treatment is systematically applied across settings, therapists, and time.

Treatments developed and conducted under remote or contrived conditions risk a second threat to generalization and maintenance. They often overlook the functional properties of natural situations on clients' behavior. By developing and conducting treatment in the course of the client's usual environment and activities, it is possible to identify conditions that affect the client positively or negatively and to incorporate this information into the treatment regime. In particular, the probability of successful generalization and maintenance of improvement rests heavily on correcting the natural conditions and contingencies provoking and reinforcing problems. In short, treatment developed and conducted in the natural environment facilitates behavioral generalization and maintenance, in part by increasing the likelihood that it is realistic and replicable across situations and time, and in part by enabling treatment that rearranges natural, functional environmental conditions, particularly the correction of those features maintaining the problem.

Although treatment should be geared to the natural environment whenever possible, in some cases it is not practical or effective to begin intervention in that context. The degree of departure from usual practice and prevailing conditions ranges widely. With dangerous and highly disruptive behavior problems, clients may have to be assigned special staff or be served in special treatment environments until behavior is improved. Such extreme measures are relatively rare. However, it often becomes necessary to employ elements of initial treatment that are contrived, intensive, or otherwise depart from usual practice. For example, in order to establish appropriate social behavior, it may be necessary to use edible or other "artificial" reinforcers at extremely high frequencies (e.g., every 1–2 minutes). Clearly, procedures such as this cannot be continued for extended periods, but nevertheless may be necessary to produce initial behavior change. This volume and other literature describe a host of means of maintaining gains following initial treatment with intensive or contrived procedures (Barton, Brulle, & Repp, 1986; Drabman, Hammer, & Rosenbaum, 1979; Koegel & Rincover, 1977; Mank & Horner, 1987; Walker & Buckley, 1972). These include:

Successively thinning reinforcement from continuous to intermittent schedules
Increasing the delay between a behavior and its reinforcement (or between a
    token and its exchange)
Shifting from contrived to naturally occurring reinforcement (e.g., from food
    to socials)
Shifting from contrived to more natural consequences for the problem (e.g.,
    from a token fine to a reprimand)
Fading out highly structured, therapist-controlled conditions and contingencies
    to, for example, honor systems and other types of self-control and peer-
    support programs
Fading in realistic conditions and situations (e.g., training demands) that had
    provoked problem behavior and were thus abridged during initial treatment

These examples illustrate the variety of means that may aid in maintaining gains across environments and times. Although it is essential to move to practical and natural procedures, the following cautions, based more on clinical experience than data, bear consideration:

1. The point at which it is decided to begin the transition from intense treatment to maintenance procedures may affect success. If fading and thinning begin following a brief and variable period of improvement, all effects may be lost. Improvement must be solid and relatively stable before changes are made. On the other hand, it may be possible to keep initial treatment in place too long, such that the slightest omission or alteration will disrupt improvement. The latter outcome seems particularly likely in treatment featuring intensive coverage and reinforcement, where clients may resist reductions in their level and even regress to previous levels.

2. The *rate* of change may also be crucial. It is standard to recommend that transitions across procedures and parameters be made gradually, and that the rate of change and size of steps be adjusted to the client's behavior. However, few empirically derived guidelines exist. In actual practice, one often sees the rate of change dictated by other factors, such as pressure to move on to another "squeeky wheel" or the availability of extra personnel for only a brief time. With such rapid and capricious transitions, behavioral improvement may not be sustained.

3. The *extent* of change represents a third consideration. Fading, thinning, and substituting procedures can only be stretched to a point. In some cases, maintenance regimes appear to be selected on the basis of appearances and compatibility with the philosophy and practice of the overall program, but may contain no clinically functional procedures for the individual. It is certainly possible that problem behavior can be successfully maintained under conditions and contingencies that are natural and normalized, but in some cases these procedures and parameters will not be sufficient to sustain improvement. In these instances, function should take precedence over appearance or philosophy. If, for example, social reinforcers fail to sustain appropriate alternative behavior, then edible reinforcers may continue to be necessary until alternative reinforcers are developed. In a similar manner, all procedural changes (e.g., scheduling delays and intermittency in reinforcement, fading conditions in and out, and substituting one consequence for another) can only be justified if they are effective in maintaining improvement. Instead, problem behavior too often reemerges under maintenance regimes that are defined procedurally, not functionally.

In general, through careful development and conduct of initial treatment and through equally careful changes in that treatment, the likelihood of generalization and maintenance can be enhanced. Although it may be possible to obtain pervasive, durable improvement with procedures that are natural, economical, and normalized, one must expect and prepare for cases where it is not.

With longstanding and intractable problem behavior, it is very possible that improvement will deteriorate without some degree and type of *systematic* maintenance regime *continued indefinitely*. Clinical experience suggests that even after sustained periods of little or no problem, the behavior remains in the individual's repertoire, ready to reemerge when conditions and contingencies again provoke and reinforce it relative to more appropriate patterns of responding. In a real sense, our attention spans must match or exceed those of our clients, ensuring that we remember problems the client is capable of displaying and remain vigilant in arranging conditions that maintain improvement in them.

ORGANIZING AND MANAGING THE LIVING ENVIRONMENT

The preceding section described a sampling of means by which generalization and maintenance may be programmed, as well as cautions about the limits within which such methods may be successful. As has been suggested, failures in generalizing and maintaining improvement may indicate that the procedures and parameters have been pushed beyond a level the client can tolerate. In fact, such failures too often point to the fact that clinical procedures have been discontinued altogether. The issue is not poor generalization and maintenance of *effects*, but poor maintenance of *effort;* shortfalls may rest less on the failure of technology than on its lack of use. The problems of ensuring that intervention is applied correctly and consistently in all situations and over time are universally acknowledged. However, the reasons for and possible approaches to these problems are often ignored.

In reviewing facilities and programs serving clients with severe problem behavior, it becomes clear that in some cases too much is being attempted simultaneously. In contrast to years past, many programs could now benefit from rank ordering and delimiting their priorities, defining what they can and should do first and well before adding additional goals (Judith Favell, Favell, Riddle, & Risley, 1984). In programs treating severe behavior problems, for example, training in alternate appropriate behavior such as communication and social skills would be addressed as the highest priority, preempting, if necessary, training in all other areas until these alternatives to problem behavior are well-developed (see Carr, Chapter 10, for elaboration). Furthermore, in such programs the introduction of any new priority, including the training of new skills, would be referenced against whether the previously learned skills could be properly maintained. For instance, if adding new self-help training programs in the morning would disrupt caregivers' ability to encourage and respond to ongoing appropriate behavior and to arrange activities that control low rates of problem behavior, then the self-help programs would need to be rescheduled to another time.

In general, if the introduction of new priorities disrupts generalization and maintenance regimes, then these new goals and activities should be delayed until both can be done in a high-quality fashion. Such an approach is rational, given the futility of trying to train/treat too many behaviors at one time, the fact that generalization and maintenance activities require time and attention (i.e., they do not slip naturally and effortlessly into the normal course of activities), and the waste in losing arduously gained skills, especially when their loss results in the reemergence of behavior problems.

Despite this logic, generalization and maintenance efforts are often not considered a high priority, but instead are overshadowed by a predominance on behavior *change*. Habilitation and educational plans tend to focus on teaching new skills and treating problems; little credit or reimbursement is paid for generalizing and maintaining those gains. This preoccupation often means that necessary conditions and contingencies are not arranged to ensure pervasive, durable improvement. Caregivers must have the time and be expected to arrange opportunities for appropriate behavior to occur and to respond to problems in prescribed ways. Similarly, conditions and contingencies must be arranged to ensure that caregivers learn these skills quickly and proficiently and perform them consistently across days, weeks, months, and years (James Favell, Favell, & Risley, 1981). These issues point to the need to attend to a variety of factors well beyond the technology of treatment, generalization and maintenance of behavior problems per se. These factors are discussed in the remaining subsections of this chapter.

Service Orchestration

Habilitation plans (individualized habilitation plans, or IHPs, and individualized education programs, or IEPs) typically contain precise and detailed descriptions of methods used in teaching skills and treating problems (Reid, Parsons, & Schepis, 1986). They often include far less information on how generalization and maintenance should be programmed. In programs for treating behavior problems, this is of particular concern because treatment cannot be scheduled, but must occur whenever and wherever appropriate and inappropriate behavior occurs. What is needed are detailed protocols of how to incorporate treatment procedures in the normal course of activities and in the context of the usual realities. This dearth points to the need for more detailed and reality-tested habilitation plans (Reid et al., 1986). Just as important, such plans must be translated into functional schedules of both client and staff activities across all settings and times (Jones, Favell, & Risley, 1983). The schedules should be devised so that there is time to ensure not only training but generalization and maintenance activities as well. These schedules must be developed through actual experience in the normal course of activities and must incorporate contingency plans for such realities as medical emergencies and differing levels of staff. Such realistically devised schedules serve as a basis for ensuring that all important activities are conducted, by reflecting careful planning and orchestration of activities, by prompting staff adherence to those tasks, and by enabling supervisory monitoring of that compliance, all of which are essential to making certain that staff provide a consistent opportunity for clients to display and be positively reinforced for appropriate behavior, which is the essence of generalizing and maintaining improvement.

Staff Training

Clearly, staff need to learn skills in teaching, treating, generalizing, and maintaining improvements in their clients' behavior. In many cases, variability and regression in clients can be attributed to staff who do not know what to expect, how to encourage clients' adaptive skills, or how to respond to their inappropriate behavior. Although effective staff training is essential, it must be matched by the need for *efficiency* in training (Page, Iwata, & Reid, 1982). Staff need to be taught necessary skills in a minimum amount of time and with minimal disruption to client services.

Efficiency is stressed not only for its obvious virtues but because *inefficient* staff training constitutes an actual disruption of client services. In order to provide consistent. high-quality services, staff must be knowledgeable about and fully equipped to meet clients' needs. However, many staff training efforts remove staff from clients at times that reduce needed coverage and services, and for lengthy periods of time. The training is often time-consuming because it includes information that may be helpful but is not essential in performing the most important aspects of the job. Not only may skills and information be less than relevant to work expectancies, but even essential skills trained often do not transfer to the workplace when they have been taught under conditions that are removed and dissimilar from that natural setting.

Sources of inefficiency must be reduced if consistent, high-quality services are to be provided. It should be realistic to expect that with reasonable screening and clear definition of roles, new staff can learn the *essentials* of their job in a relatively short period (Risley & Favell, 1979). Although this time would not be sufficient to instruct staff in elaborate and complex teaching procedures, it should be adequate to teach staff how to set the occasion for and reinforce ongoing appropriate behavior, which is essential to generalization and maintenance of improvement in problems.

Staff Supervision

Because successful generalization and maintenance rests on ensuring that clients' programs are carried out correctly and consistently across settings and over time, variability and drift in staff performance represent serious threats to such efforts. New treatment and training programs are often adhered to scrupulously, but as the novelty fades, as priorities shift, and as behavior problems improve, there is a tendency to alter or omit procedures that are crucial to continued improvement. Although a variety of factors may be implicated in this problem, it commonly reflects the need for improved staff supervison (Reid & Whitman, 1983). Many programs suffer from such problems, and do not adequately select, train, enable, or expect managers to properly supervise their staff. Without adequate supervision, staff performance usually strays, often in undesirable directions, and client behavior correspondingly deteriorates.

Research literature and actual experience point to means of enhancing staff performance through improved supervisory practices. Fundamentally, this involves frequent, on-site monitoring of clearly specified dimensions of staff performance followed by differential positive and corrective feedback (e.g., Reid & Shoemaker, 1984). Although obvious and clearly effective, such aspects of supervision are often neglected. In some cases, "simple" procedures such as giving feedback prove to be difficult to teach and learn. Perhaps more commonly, these practices are learned, but gradually disappear for the same

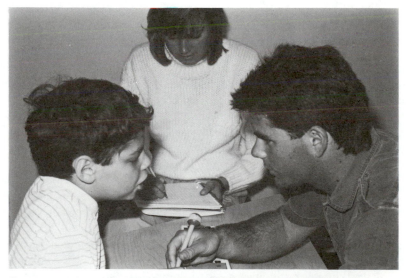

Frequent on-site monitoring and feedback from supervisors improves the quality of instruction.

reasons staff performance drifts. Supervisory behavior is maintained by procedures similar to those successful in maintaining staff behavior. Unless monitoring and feedback are identified as top priorities, and unless the supervisor is evaluated and given feedback on his or her extent of compliance with this standard, it is likely that such practices will disappear in the crush of paperwork and other priorities. In short, successful generalization and maintenance of behavioral improvement in clients rests on staff responding properly and consistently, which in turn depends on consistent, on-site supervision. Where these practices are not expected and reinforced, poor generalization and maintenance of client, staff, and supervisory behavior can be expected.

Staff Withdrawal

As indicated, consistency and quality of treatment services rests on the presence of adequate numbers of properly trained staff. Variability in training personnel can slow and disrupt progress in initial treatment phases, but perhaps has even more deleterious effects on generalization and maintenance efforts. High and unpredictable rates of absenteeism cause extreme problems in compliance to schedules and regimes. Under conditions of less than optimal coverage, perhaps some of the first staff behaviors to deteriorate are those that are most pivotal to successful generalization and maintenance: prompting and reinforcing appropriate behavior and responding to problems in prescribed ways in the natural course of activities. Considering the importance of staff attendance to the continuity and quality of services, and given widespread problems in this area (Zaharia & Baumeister, 1978), this issue warrants serious attention. Research is revealing promising methods of controlling absenteeism, through reinforcing good attendance with lottery participation (Iwata, Bailey, Brown, Foshee, & Alpern, 1976), group contingencies (Reid, Schuh-Wear, & Brannon, 1978), and other means (Shoemaker & Reid, 1980). Through such methods, staff attendance, a crucial element in ensuring pervasive and durable improvement in clients, can be improved.

An equally serious and widespread threat to proper and consistent treatment is staff turnover. The loss of information and the problem of inconsistency caused by constant staff rotation through a program can be a major disruption to generalizing and maintaining improvement. Maintenance regimes for problem behavior may be particularly susceptible to deterioration, because neither their presence nor need may be obvious to new staff, given that the problem is occurring at a low rate.

In the authors' experience, turnover can be reduced through such means as modifying hiring and orientation procedures and improving work conditions. Nevertheless, turnover will always exist in programs involving such difficult work. However, steps can be taken to offset the negative impact of this flux. For example, recording systems and staff training can be streamlined so that new staff can quickly retrieve and learn information on the most essential parts of the job. At present, most client records discourage rather than facilitate information retrieval. With patience, one may locate current treatment and training programs, but finding information on how previously targeted skills and behaviors are generalized and maintained is typically very difficult. It is relatively easy to organize this information in a clear and accessible fashion, a step that is essential if continuity of programming with high staff turnover is to be assured.

Further, as turnover increases, the need for efficiency in staff training correspondingly increases. Fortunately, improved efficiency need not decrease effectiveness, within limits. Checklists describing elements of how to conduct a leisure activity, how to give a bath, or how to prompt and reinforce appropriate social behavior can replace the lengthy and complex narratives that are often found in written plans and programs. *In situ* training based on these simple and clear checklists can equal or exceed the effectiveness of lengthier didactic instruction (Lattimore, Stephens, Favell, & Risley, 1984).

These brief examples hint at the innumerable ways to address problems such as staff withdrawal that affect generalization and maintenance efforts. Clearly the list of problems described here has not been exhaustive; the problems illustrate, however, how generalization and maintenance of improvement may be influenced by countless dimensions beyond the scope of the technology of intervention. The emphasis of service delivery systems (and their funding sources) must be clearly focused on a manageable array of priorities in order to elevate generalization and maintenance to a level of significance comparable to or greater than initial treatment and training. Research on treatment technology must be matched with investigations and applications of methods to improve service orchestration, staff training, staff supervision, and staff withdrawal. Advances in these areas will most surely have as important an impact on generalization and maintenance as any technological advances.

REFERENCES

Azrin, N.H., & Holz, W.C. (1966). Punishment. In W.K. Honig (Ed.), *Operant behavior: Areas of research and application* (pp. 380–447). New York: Appleton-Century-Crofts.

Baer, D.M. (1981). *How to plan for generalization*. Austin, TX: PRO-ED.

Baer, D.M., & Wolf, M.M. (1970). The entry into natural communities of reinforcement. In R. Ulrich, T. Stachnik, & J. Mabry (Eds.), *Control of human behavior: From cure to prevention* (pp. 319–324). Glenview, IL: Scott, Foresman.

Barton, L.E., Brulle, A.R., & Repp, A.C. (1986). Maintenance of therapeutic change by momentary DRO. *Journal of Applied Behavior Analysis, 19,* 277–282.

Birnbrauer, J.S. (1968). Generalization of punishment effects: A case study. *Journal of Applied Behavior Analysis, 1,* 201–211.

Carr, E.G. (1977). The motivation of self-injurious behavior: A review of some hypotheses. *Psychological Bulletin, 84*, 800–816.

Carr, E.G., & Durand, V.M. (1985). Reducing behavior problems through functional communication training. *Journal of Applied Behavior Analysis, 18*, 111–126.

Carr, E.G., Newsom, C.D., & Binkoff, J.A. (1980). Escape as a factor in the aggressive behavior of two retarded children. *Journal of Applied Behavior Analysis, 13*, 101–117.

Dietz, D.E.D., & Repp, A.C. (1983). Reducing behavior through reinforcement. *Exceptional Education Quarterly, 3*, 34–46.

Drabman, R.S., Hammer, D., & Rosenbaum, M.S. (1979). Assessing generalization in behavior modification with children: The generalization map. *Behavioral assessment, 1*, 203–219.

Eason, L.J., White, M.J., & Newsom, C. (1982). Generalized reduction of self-stimulatory behavior: An effect of teaching appropriate play to autistic children. *Analysis and Intervention in Developmental Disabilities, 2*, 157–169.

Favell, James E., Favell, Judith E., & Risley, T.R. (1981). A quality-assurance system for ensuring client rights in mental retardation facilities. In G.T. Hannah, W.P. Christian, & H.B. Clark (Eds.), *Preservation of client rights: A handbook for practitioners providing therapeutic, educational, and rehabilitative services*. New York: Free Press.

Favell, Judith E. (Chairperson), Azrin, N.H., Baumeister, A.A., Carr, E.G., Dorsey, M.F., Forehand, R., Foxx, R.M., Lovaas, O.I., Rincover, A., Risley, T.R., Romanczyk, R.G., Russo, D.C., Schroeder, S.R., & Solnick, J.V. (1982). The treatment of self-injurious behavior [Monograph]. *Behavior Therapy, 13*, 529–554.

Favell, Judith E., Favell, James E., Riddle, J.I., & Risley, T.R. (1984). Promoting change in mental retardation facilities: Getting services from the paper to the people. In W.P. Christian, G.T. Hannah, & T.J. Glahn (Eds.), *Programming effective human services: Strategies for institutional change and client transition*. New York: Plenum.

Favell, Judith E., McGimsey, J.F., & Schell, R.M. (1982). Treatment of self-injury by providing alternate sensory activities. *Analysis and Intervention in Developmental Disabilities, 2*, 83–104.

Foxx, R.M., & Livesay, J. (1984). Maintenance of response suppression following overcorrection: A 10-year retrospective examination of eight cases. *Analysis and Intervention in Developmental Disabilities, 4*, 65–79.

Iwata, B.A., Bailey, J.S., Brown, K.M., Foshee, T.J., & Alpern, M. (1976). A performance-based lottery to improve residential care and training by institutional staff. *Journal of Applied Behavior Analysis, 9*, 417–431.

Iwata, B.A., Dorsey, M.F., Slifer, K.J., Bauman, K.E., & Richman, G.S. (1982). Toward a functional analysis of self-injury. *Analysis and Intervention in Developmental Disabilities, 2*, 3–20.

Jones, M.L., Favell, J.E., & Risley, T.R. (1983). Socioecological programming of the mentally retarded. In J.L. Matson & F. Andrasik (Eds.), *Treatment issues and innovations in mental retardation*. New York: Plenum.

Journal of Applied Behavior Analysis. (1968–1985). *Behavior analysis in developmental disabilities: 1968-1985* (Reprint series, Vol. 1).

Kazdin, A.E., & Esveldt-Dawson, K. (1981). *How to maintain behavior.* Austin, TX: PRO-ED.

Koegel, R.L., & Rincover, A. (1977). Research on the difference between generalization and maintenance in extra-therapy responding. *Journal of Applied Behavior Analysis, 10,* 1–12.

Lattimore, J., Stephens, T.E., Favell, J.E., & Risley, T.R. (1984). Increasing direct care staff compliance to individualized physical therapy body positioning prescriptions: Prescriptive checklists. *Mental Retardation, 22,* 79–84.

LaVigna, G.W., & Donnellan, A.M. (1986). *Alternatives to punishment: Solving behavior problems with non-aversive strategies.* New York: Irvington.

Lovaas, O.I., & Favell, J.E. (in press). Protection for clients undergoing aversive/restrictive interventions. *Education and Treatment of Children* (spec. issue).

Lovaas, O.I., Freitag, G., Gold, V.J., & Kassorla, I.C. (1965). Experimental studies in childhood schizophrenia: Analysis of self-destructive behavior. *Journal of Experimental Child Psychology, 2,* 67–84.

Lovaas, O.I., Koegel, R., Simmons, J.Q., & Long, J.S. (1973). Some generalization and follow-up measures on autistic children in behavior therapy. *Journal of Applied Behavior Analysis, 6,* 131–166.

Lovaas, O.I., & Simmons, J.Q. (1969). Manipulation of self-destruction in three retarded children. *Journal of Applied Behavior Analysis, 2,* 143–157.

Mank, D.M., & Horner, R.H. (1987). Self-recruited feedback: A cost-effective procedure for maintaining behavior. *Research in Developmental Disabilities, 8,* 91–112.

Page, T.J., Iwata, B.A., & Reid, D.H. (1982). Pyramidal training: A large-scale application with institutional staff. *Journal of Applied Behavior Analysis, 15,* 335–351.

Parrish, J.M., Cataldo, M.F., Kolko, D.J., Neef, N.A., & Egel, A.L. (1986). Experimental analysis of response covariation among compliant and inappropriate behaviors. *Journal of Applied Behavior Analysis, 19,* 241–254.

Reid, D.H., Parsons, M.B., & Schepis, M.M. (1986). Treatment planning and implementation. In F.J. Fuoco & W.P. Christian (Eds.), *Behavior analysis and therapy in residential programs* (pp. 50–75). New York: Van Nostrand Reinhold.

Reid, D.H., Schuh-Wear, C.L., & Brannon, M.E. (1978). Use of a group contingency to decrease staff absenteeism in a state institution. *Behavior Modification, 2,* 251–266.

Reid, D.H., & Shoemaker, J. (1984). Behavioral supervision: Methods of improving institutional staff performance. In W.P. Christian, G.T. Hannah, & Glahn, T.J. (Eds.), *Programming effective human services: Strategies for institutional change and client transition* (pp. 39–61). New York: Plenum.

Reid, D.H., & Whitman, T.L. (1983). Behavorial staff management in institutions: A critical review of effectiveness and acceptability. *Analysis and Intervention in Developmental Disabilities, 3,* 131–149.

Rincover, A., Cook, R., Peoples, A., & Packard, D. (1979). Sensory extinction and sensory reinforcement principles for programming multiple adaptive behavior change. *Journal of Applied Behavior Analysis, 12,* 221–233.

Risley, T.R., & Favell, J.E. (1979). Constructing a living environment in an institution. In L. Hamerlynck (Ed.), *Behavioral systems for the developmentally disabled: II. Institutional, clinic, and community environments.* New York: Brunner/Mazel.

Schroeder, S.R., Kanoy, R.C., Mulick, J.A., Rojahn, J., Thios, S.J., Stephens, M., & Hawk, B. (1982). Environmental antecedents which affect management and maintenance of programs for self-injurious behavior. In J.H. Hollis & C.E. Meyers (Eds.), *Life-threatening behavior: Analysis and intervention* (pp. 105–159). Washington, DC: American Association on Mental Deficiency.

Shoemaker, J., & Reid, D.H. (1980). Decreasing chronic absenteeism among institutional staff: Effects of a low-cost attendance program. *Journal of Organizational Behavior Management, 2,* 317–328.

Stokes, T.F., & Baer, D.M. (1977). An implicit technology of generalization. *Journal of Applied Behavior Analysis, 10,* 349–367.

Touchette, P.E., MacDonald, R.F., & Langer, S.N. (1985). A scatter plot for identifying stimulus control of problem behavior. *Journal of Applied Behavior Analysis, 18,* 343–351.

Walker, H.M., & Buckley, N.K. (1972). Programming generalization and maintenance of treatment effects across time and across settings. *Journal of Applied Behavior Analysis, 5,* 209–224.

Whitman, T.L., Scibak, J.W., & Reid, D.H. (Eds.) (1983). *Behavior modification with the severely and profoundly retarded: Research and application.* New York: Academic Press.

Zaharia, E.S., & Baumeister, A.A. (1978). Technician turnover and absenteeism in public residential facilities. *American Journal of Mental Deficiency, 82,* 580–593.

Chapter 9

The Effect of Competing Behavior on the Generalization and Maintenance of Adaptive Behavior in Applied Settings

Robert H. Horner and Felix F. Billingsley

The role of competing stimulus control relationships on the generalization and maintenance of adaptive behavior is discussed in this chapter. The concept of "competing behavior" expands behavioral analysis to address more adequately the complexity of applied settings. In contrast to contrived laboratory environments, learners in applied settings often face multiple stimuli that are discriminative for different responses. At any single time, the stimulus control relationships associated with different stimuli may be in competition. Understanding how these competing relationships develop and affect responding is of major concern for an applied technology of generalization. A learner who has acquired a new, adaptive skill may demonstrate excellent generalization across new situations until a new situation is presented that contains a strong competing stimulus. The competing stimulus is likely to elicit an old, undesirable be-

The activity that is the subject of this report was supported in whole or in part by the U.S. Department of Education, Contract 300-82-0362 and Contract 300-82-0364. However, the opinions expressed herein do not necessarily reflect the position or policy of the U.S. Department of Education, and no official endorsement by the department should be inferred.

The authors extend sincere appreciation to Drs. Kathleen Liberty, Robert L. Koegel, Richard W. Albin, and Susan Epps for their helpful comments on early drafts of this chapter.

havior. The practical effect is that the new, adaptive response does not general-ize to that situation. The reason for this result is not, however, a simple lack of generalization but inadequate stimulus control to overcome the old, competing response.

The problem of competing behaviors is seen often by parents who teach their children table manners. A child may have experienced several years of whining or grabbing as the functional response for getting desired food items. Upon reaching a certain socially appropriate age, new food-requesting skills are taught. Often, however, asking politely is a less efficient method of getting food, and the old responses of whining or grabbing may occur even though the child is capable of polite requesting. In this example, whining or grabbing are competing responses that are under strong stimulus control, and are performed instead of the desired response.

One reason adaptive behavior may fail to generalize or be maintained is because the new behavior is masked by older, stronger, competing responses. This is an important concept for describing why behaviors may generalize to some new situations and not to others, and why a behavior that has been main-tained well for an extended time may suddenly deteriorate (Marholin & Tou-chette, 1979). This chapter: 1) provides a structure for analyzing generalization and maintenance problems that arise as a function of competing stimulus con-trol relationships, 2) suggests implications for applied intervention when com-peting behaviors exist, and 3) provides recommendations for applied research on competing behaviors that will increase the precision of our technology for achieving generalization and maintenance.

A STRUCTURE FOR
ANALYZING COMPETING BEHAVIORS

When a new skill is learned to criterion, the learner acquires the physical ability to perform the target responses, and those responses are brought under appro-priate stimulus control. A response is under stimulus control when presentation of a stimulus reliably changes the probability of that response (Terrace, 1966). The stimulus control developed during instruction has life-style impact when the new skill generalizes and is maintained. More specifically, the new skill should: 1) be performed across the full range of "appropriate" stimulus situa-tions the learner encounters as part of his or her day-to-day activity (new peo-ple, places, and materials); 2) *not* be performed in "inappropriate," nontrained situations; and 3) be maintained over time (Horner, Bellamy, & Colvin, 1984).

This analysis emphasizes that it is the controlling relationship between stimuli and responses that generalizes to nontrained situations and is main-tained across time. When a behavior is referred to as "generalizing," what is meant is that the stimulus control over that behavior generalizes to some non-trained stimulus or situation. When a behavior is referred to as "maintaining," what is meant is that a stimulus control relationship is stable or consistent across time. The role of stimulus control within generalization and mainte-nance suggests two important factors that are critical for understanding the role that competing behaviors play in creating generalization and maintenance prob-lems. The first is defining the set of situations that are expected to control the desirable behavior (the instructional universe), and the second is differentiation of the stimuli in a situation that should and should not control the desired be-havior (i.e., relevant versus irrelevant stimuli).

Instructional Universe

The instructional universe defines a group of situations (stimuli), all of which control the target response (Becker, Engelmann, & Thomas, 1975; Engelmann & Carnine, 1982). A person who learns to cross streets, for example, may be expected to generalize across the instructional universe "all streets in town" when the skill is acquired. The instructional universe includes trained and non-trained situations. In Figure 1, the set of stimuli inside the circle are members of

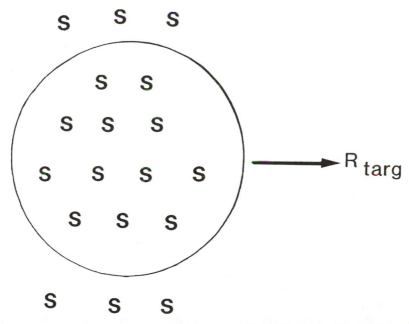

Figure 1. Instructional universe for target response (R_{targ}). All stimuli within the circle are members of the instructional universe (relevant) and should control R_{targ}. All stimuli outside the circle are irrelevant and should not affect R_{targ}.

the instructional universe. Any one of them should control the target response, R_{targ}. The stimuli outside the circle are not members of the instructional universe, and should be irrelevant with respect to R_{targ}. Defining the instructional universe is functional both for designing instructional programs focused on generalized skills (Albin, McDonnell, & Wilcox, 1987: Billingsley, 1984; Horner, McDonnell, & Bellamy, 1986), and for assessment of generalization and maintenance problems after instruction (Horner et al., 1984). Among the most useful aspects of the instructional universe is the opportunity it provides for clearly defining those stimuli that are "relevant" versus those that are "irrelevant."

Relevant versus Irrelevant Stimuli

Relevant stimuli are those that change the likelihood of a target response. An objective of teaching is to bring adaptive behaviors under control of appropriate, relevant stimuli, and not under control of irrelevant stimuli (e.g., "say /b/ in the presence of 'b' but not 'd' "). Generalization errors often are attributed to the learner failing to respond to what should be a relevant stimulus, or treating what should be an irrelevant stimulus as if it were relevant (Horner, Albin, & Ralph, 1986; Horner et al., 1984; Horner, Williams, & Stevely, 1987; McDonnell & Horner, 1985). Maintenance errors are often attributed to relevant stimuli losing stimulus control over time. In both cases the source of the errors may be less a function of changes in the stimulus control exerted by relevant stimuli, and more a function of competing responses masking adaptive behavior (Billingsley & Neel, 1985; Horner, Albin, & Mank, 1986).

Competing Behavior

Competing behaviors are responses that occur at the expense of targeted responses. A competing behavior typically has a different topography from the target response, and a learning history that is separate from the target (adaptive) response. Competing behaviors are aptly named. They occur in place of, or at the desired time for, targeted, adaptive responses. Researchers interested in the theoretical analysis of generalization and maintenance have recognized that the presence of competing stimuli may block or overshadow the acquisition of new skills (Honig & Urcuioli, 1981; Kamin, 1968; Newman & Baron, 1965). Little theoretical work has been done, however, analyzing the effects of competing stimuli, and the behaviors they control, on generalization after the target behavior is learned. This process, labeled "masking," recognizes that stimulus control relationships developed prior to instruction may reduce the array of situations to which a new skill will generalize or be maintained (Honig & Urcuioli, 1981; Mackintosh, 1977; Rudolph, Honig, & Gerry, 1969). In this way, theoretical analyses emphasize the complex interactions that occur when multiple controlling stimuli are presented (cf., Schreibman, Chapter 2). One of the great disadvantages of applied settings is the difficulty in defining exactly which stimulus (or stimuli) controls a behavior. This problem is more easily addressed in the managed environment of an operant chamber.

In applied settings, it is recognized that the addition of competing stimuli may inhibit the maintenance of an otherwise stable behavior, or that the presence of competing stimuli in a nontrained setting may reduce the likelihood of generalization of an adaptive skill to that setting (Horner, Albin, & Mank, 1986). Applied researchers have been extremely interested in understanding the variables that affect competing behavior. Analysis of research undertaken to date suggests four types of situations in which competing behaviors affect generalization and/or maintenance. The four situation types are created by attending first to whether the discriminative stimuli for the target (desirable) and competing (undesirable) responses are the same or different and then by determining if the reinforcers for the target and competing responses are the same or different. A diagram of the four problem situations that result is provided in Figure 2, and discussed in detail next.

Situation A: Different S^Ds, Same Reinforcers   The first situation in which competing behaviors may affect generalization and maintenance is when the competing behavior is: 1) controlled by some "irrelevant" stimulus (S_{comp}) that is different from, but present with, the target discriminative stimulus (S_{targ}) and 2) results in access to the same reinforcer as the target behavior. McDonnell, Horner, and Williams (1984) report an example of this situation in which four high school–age students with severe mental retardation were trained to deliver the correct number of dollars to a cashier when purchasing items from stores with checkout counters. In the classroom, under simulated

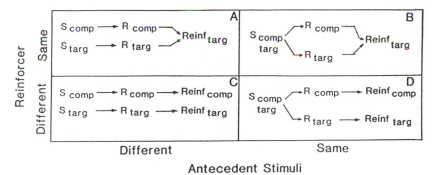

Figure 2. Competing behavior analysis. S_{comp} = discriminative stimulus for competing response; S_{targ} = discriminative stimulus for target response; R_{comp} = competing response; R_{targ} = target response; $Reinf_{comp}$ = reinforcer maintaining competing response; $Reinf_{targ}$ = reinforcer maintaining target response (or target response *and* competing response).

conditions, the students paid with fluency and competence. In actual stores, however, two students reverted to an old response of simply handing all money to the cashier rather than counting out the correct dollar amount. It was hypothesized that "handing over all money" was a competing response under control of stimuli existing in the actual stores, and led to the same reinforcer (obtaining items) as performing the targeted, paying response. When training was extended beyond the classroom to community stores, and included instruction on "not handing over all money," there was an increase in the use of correct payment responses in nontrained stores.

Situation B: Same S^{D}s, Same Reinforcers   The second situation in which competing behaviors may affect generalization and maintenance occurs when the competing behavior is under control of a stimulus that is a member of the targeted instructional universe, and results in access to the same reinforcer as the target behavior. Billingsley and Neel (1985) report an example of this situation with two 8-year-olds with severe mental retardation. Both students were nonverbal, and consistently grabbed for food during lunch. Even after being trained to use manual signs to indicate desired food items, the competing behavior of grabbing remained at a high frequency in generalization and maintenance situations. The discriminative stimulus of food (within grabbing range) had strong control over grabbing and resulted in access to food. When the authors prevented grabbing from resulting in food access, both students increased their use of manual signs and decreased their use of grabbing. O'Brien, Azrin, and Bugle (1972) document a similar example with young children who were taught to walk instead of crawl. Four children with profound mental retardation were taught to walk. In two cases, however, the children walked with substantial difficulty and were more likely to use their fluent and effective strategy of crawling to get from one place to another. Only when these two children were restrained from getting anywhere when they crawled, did walking become their common mode of locomotion. In both of these studies the authors suggested that the competing behavior not only had a strong history of reinforcement but may have been an easier strategy to enable the students to achieve the desired outcome. By decreasing the effectiveness of the competing behavior to produce the reinforcer, there was a significant increase in the likelihood of the preferred target response.

Situation C: Different S^{D}s, Different Reinforcers   The third situation in which competing behaviors may affect generalization and maintenance is when the competing behavior is under control of a nontrained stimulus and produces a reinforcer different from the target reinforcer. The discriminative stimuli for both the target response (R_{targ}) and the competing response (R_{comp}) are present. R_{targ} will lead to the target reinforcer ($Reinf_{comp}$), and R_{comp} will lead to the competing reinforcer ($Reinf_{comp}$). If the competing reinforcer is more powerful than the target reinforcer, there is a high likelihood that R_{comp} will be performed. Solomon and Wahler (1973) describe a classic example of this situation with 10 "disruptive" sixth graders. The authors observed "positive" and "disruptive" behavior in the classroom setting. They hypothesized that positive classroom behavior was evoked by teacher requests and maintained by teacher attention, and that disruptive behavior was evoked by peer prompts and was maintained by peer attention. When given an assignment (S_{targ}) to be done with other students (S_{comp}), these youngsters were very likely to engage in disruptive behavior. The authors reduced access to $Reinf_{comp}$ and increased access to $Reinf_{targ}$ by training other students in the classroom to ignore disruptive behavior and to attend to positive behavior. Following the intervention, there was a dramatic reduction in disruptive behavior, and a concomitant increase in adaptive behavior.

Situation D: Same S^Ds, Different Reinforcers   The final situation in which competing behaviors may affect generalization and maintenance occurs when the competing behavior is controlled by a stimulus within the instructional universe, and is maintained by a reinforcer different from the target reinforcer. An adaptive behavior may generalize to many nontrained situations, but may fail to generalize to some situations that already have a history of controlling a competing behavior. Compliance with requests, for example, may be developed with a teacher, and may generalize to an array of other people. When the student's parents deliver a request, however, a prior history with non-compliance may mask the training, and previously learned aggressive or escape behaviors may occur. Engelmann and Colvin (1983) described this pattern with several students identified with severe behavior disorders. In each case additional training was necessary within those situations in the instructional universe that already exerted strong control over competing behavior.

This final situation has also been documented in reports focusing on self-injurious behavior. Carr and Durand (1985a, 1985b) detail multiple accounts in which youngsters with autism engaged in the competing behaviors of head hitting, scratching, or biting rather than performing adaptive behaviors that were in their repertoire. In several instances the competing reinforcer of escaping the situation through a self-injurious response was hypothesized as more powerful than the praise and/or edibles for performing the target skill. Eliminating the escape function of the self-injurious behavior resulted in substantial increases in the target response. A complete discussion of this pattern is provided by Carr in Chapter 10 of this text.

Complex Analysis of Competing Behavior

The preceding analysis of competing behavior emphasizes that natural settings continually present stimuli within concurrent schedule formats. The analysis focuses on the importance of prior learning histories as a mechanism by which strong, competing behaviors are built, potentially inhibiting the generalization and/or maintenance of desired behaviors. Although the scope of this chapter does not allow extended elaboration, at least two additional concepts should be mentioned here to expand the analysis to complex, natural settings. First, one must recognize that the natural environment often presents more than two concurrent options for responding. At any one time, a learner may be presented with stimuli that are discriminative for several different responses (indicated in Figure 3 as S_{comp_2} . . . S_{comp_n}). At present, no adequate analysis is available of how these complex, competing stimulus control relationships interact. A functional technology of generalization, especially generalized control of excess behavior, will require a much better understanding of the interaction effects under competing, concurrent conditions.

The other point to be mentioned in this analysis of competing behavior is a recognition of the role played by setting events (Leighand, 1984; Michael, 1983). Setting events do not exert direct control over responding, but modify the control exerted by other stimuli. Setting events such as fatigue or hunger may dramatically alter the probability that a target response will generalize or maintain in situations where competing relationships exist. The role of setting events is recognized in the authors' analysis, and in Figure 3, through the addi-

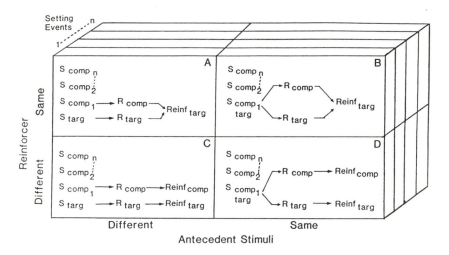

Figure 3. Competing behavior analysis with the additions of multiple competing stimuli and setting events. S_{comp} = discriminative stimulus for competing response; S_{targ} = discriminative stimulus for target response; R_{comp} = competing response; R_{targ} = target response; $Reinf_{comp}$ = reinforcer maintaining competing response; $Reinf_{targ}$ = reinforcer maintaining target response (or target response and competing response).

tion of a third dimension. The impact of setting events within the analysis of competing behavior raises again the issue of the important position played by interactions in complex natural settings. By definition, setting events are inter-action variables (Wahler & Fox, 1981). The full extent of their importance for generalization and maintenance in applied settings will become clear only as we develop the measurement and design technology needed to assess complex interactions in the natural environment.

IMPLICATIONS FOR APPLIED SETTINGS

The foregoing taxonomy of problem situations created by competing behaviors provides a structure for both assessment and intervention in applied settings.

Assessment

Stimuli in natural settings may influence behaviors that successfully compete with target skills. In addition, characteristics such as response fluency, re-sponse effort, or the likelihood of a response to produce reinforcers may affect whether target versus competing behaviors are performed in nontrained situa-tions. Current data suggest that, all things being equal, preexisting behaviors are likely to compete successfully with new behaviors if the preexisting be-haviors lead to more powerful reinforcers or more efficiently produce the same reinforcers as the target behaviors.

Conventional assessments for curriculum design emphasize the need to define the demands of current and future environments via ecological analyses (Brown et al., 1979; Falvey, 1986; Wilcox & Bellamy, 1982). When competing behaviors have been identified, however, assessment must go beyond analysis of the environmental demands, to include a more specific analysis of how the learner manages his or her environment. To develop programs with a high prob-ability of producing generalized responding, it is necessary to specify the rein-forcing functions of targeted, adaptive behaviors and determine whether stu-dents already possess alternative behaviors that effectively serve the same functions. In the event that alternative behaviors can be identified, the next step is to identify the stimuli associated with the occurrence of those behaviors in nontraining settings. It is also of value to determine whether high-probability responses exist that may not serve the same functions as target behaviors but that seem to be maintained by particularly potent reinforcers. Although sub-stantial information regarding those factors can be obtained from parents and other significant community members, a thorough assessment calls for at least a small number of pretraining observations of pupils under the natural condi-tions in which the target behaviors will be needed. Questions to be answered by such an assessment include:

1. *Does the student engage in behaviors that, although undesirable, achieve the intended result of the target behavior?* Does screaming, for instance, serve to get Carl dressed because his mother dresses him when he screams; does pinching achieve the same result (task termination) as a manual sign intended to communicate "I'm tired and want to stop now!"

2. *Where behaviors such as those just listed are noted, how efficiently and reliably do they serve the identified reinforcing function?* To answer this question, it may be reasonable to collect data on the speed with which potentially competing behaviors permit the individual to achieve the intended outcome. Liberty and Billingsley (1985) have suggested that a stopwatch be used to measure the time from the beginning of the response or response chain until the reinforcer is obtained. Concurrently, the extent to which the behavior is successful in obtaining reinforcers should be noted. (That is, do Cheryl's parents give her juice or food virtually every time she jumps up and down while flapping her hands in the middle of the living room, or do they comply with Cheryl's "request" on a more intermittent basis?)

3. *Under assessment conditions, does the pupil perform some apparently unrelated, but undesirable behavior?* (That is, does the pupil perform an undesirable behavior that does not appear to serve the reinforcing function of the target response?) For example, where the target behavior involves putting on a jacket preparatory to going outside, a pupil might engage in stereotypical behavior that appears to result in neither someone else putting the jacket on him or her nor getting to go outside. If such a behavior is noted, is that behavior observed in many other situations?

4. *Are competing behaviors correlated with the presence of some very specific stimulus (e.g., mother), or are they correlated with many general stimuli and situations?* Are controlling stimuli members of the instructional universe for the target skill, or are they irrelevant?

Intervention

Based on the outcome of pretraining assessments and subsequent observations of generalization errors and failures to obtain skill maintenance, one or a number of intervention strategies may be applied. One class of such strategies are those that may be applied within training settings, while a second class includes those that might be applied within nontraining settings (i.e., settings in which skill performance is desired, but in which training has never been conducted). Most of the strategies recommended for use in training contexts attempt to reduce the impact of competing behaviors by altering the relationship between stimuli and behavior (cf., Schroeder, Bickel, & Richmond, 1984). Those used in nontraining settings attempt to change the function of the controlling stimuli by suppressing competing behaviors or by removing the stimuli that set the occasion for those behaviors (Wolery & Gast, 1984).

Strategies within the Training Setting

Increase the Efficiency and/or Reliability of the Target Behavior   Where a competing behavior is identified that achieves the same reinforcers as the target behavior, one straightforward procedure to enhance generalization and maintenance is to ensure that the response under instruction is *at least* as equally efficient and reliable as, and preferably more so than, the competing response (Carr & Kologinsky, 1983; Horner & Budd, 1985; White, 1985). The intent here is to change the function of the controlling stimuli by providing learners with a new behavior that will be of higher priority in their behavioral repertoire than the existing behavior (cf., Bandura, 1969; Cahoon, 1968; Staddon, 1977), and that will be controlled by the same stimulus or stimuli as the existing behavior. For example, if it is found that a pupil can crawl at a rate of 70 feet per minute, an initial fluency aim for walking might be set at something beyond that rate (for a discussion of fluency aims, see White, 1985). Given a lesser aim, it would be possible for the pupil to obtain reinforcers faster by crawling than by walking. In such a case, it would not be surprising if the pupil crawled whenever the option to perform that behavior were available.

Modify, Replace, or Augment Target Behavior   Where it is improbable that the target behavior will allow the pupil to obtain reinforcers as efficiently or reliably as the competing behavior, a possible strategy is to modify, replace, or augment that behavior. For pupils with certain physical handi-

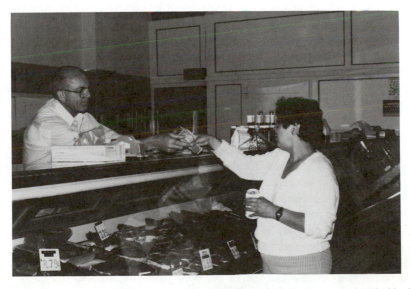

Teaching a simple purchasing skill can reduce undesirable behaviors associated with obtaining items.

caps, for example, the desired degree of fluency in walking might be unobtain-able or might require a considerable (and, perhaps, potentially damaging) expenditure of effort. In such instances, a possible strategy would be to select a different behavior to serve the particular function. If the pupil could never walk independently as fast as he or she could crawl, perhaps the use of a wheelchair or walking with a walker would be more apt to generalize and be maintained as acceptable forms of locomotion than walking independently.

As an additional illustration, a pupil (Tom) might have a very effective, though highly undesirable, way of requesting food and toys; say, head-banging. Within the home, Tom always receives food or toys when he bangs his head on the floor, the wall, or other surfaces. Because his parents never ignore the be-havior, head-banging is 100% successful in producing reinforcers. It is entirely possible that a communication program instituted at school could teach Tom manual English signs to request food or toys, but that the signs would be much easier to ignore than head-banging. Signing, therefore, would not be as suc-cessful in obtaining the desired items as the self-injurious behavior. The use of signs in the home might then rapidly disappear to be replaced by the old, highly successful head-banging behavior (Liberty & Billingsley, 1985). An appropri-ate strategy in this case might be to replace the use of manual English signs with a speech synthesis device that would be easy to activate and difficult to ignore. Alternately, the sign form might be augmented by the addition of some other behavior in order to increase its reliability. In Tom's case, he might be instructed to tap his parent's arm to get his or her attention before using the appropriate sign.

Reduce the Control Exerted by Stimuli Associated with the Competing Responses   Individuals may have in their repertoire un-desirable behaviors that successfully compete with target behaviors, not be-cause they permit acquisition of the *same* reinforcers, but because they result in *stronger* reinforcers (situations C and D in Figures 2 and 3). The third assess-ment question stated earlier is designed to elicit information regarding the na-ture of such behaviors.

If a behavior is highly generalized, in the sense that it occurs under many different situations, it is possible that the individual simply has no alternative responses in his or her repertoire to obtain reinforcers. Therefore, when new responses are learned that permit access to additional or similar forms of re-inforcement, the old behavior may occur less frequently (e.g., Carr & Kologinsky, 1983; Eason, White, & Newsom, 1982; Favell, McGimsey, & Schell, 1982). On the other hand, a frequently noted undesirable behavior could also be maintained by a particularly potent reinforcer and be one for which an acceptable and reliable alternative behavior would be difficult to identify. Where an extremely strong reinforcer maintains the behavior, therefore, it might be necessary to employ steps to suppress that behavior concurrent with the training of new responses that would permit access to other (but less potent) reinforcers. Typical suppressive measures might include practices such as extinction of brief physical restraint (Kazdin, 1980). The problem for generalization posed by the use of such methods in intervention settings is that stimuli surrounding their application may become discriminative for response suppression. For instance, a suppressive intervention could always involve the presence of a particular person (or a few known individuals), or perhaps some characteristic data-recording device such as a wrist counter. With continued exposure to the relationship between such stimuli and the intervention, it is likely that the student would come to associate application of the intervention with those stimuli and suppress the response only when they are present.

To avoid this problem, the suppressive measures should be used with a wide variety of people, places, and materials, and the measures should be paired consistently with the stimuli controlling the competing response. The objective is twofold: 1) suppress the controlling relationship between the S^D, the competing behavior, and the reinforcer for the competing behavior and 2) avoid the situation where response suppression only occurs under certain conditions. Favell and Reid provide a more complete discussion of generalized suppression in Chapter 8.

Apply General Case Methods This strategy for application within instructional contexts involves the selection and sequencing of the instructional examples, and relates to answers obtained from the fourth assessment question stated previously. It represents an extension of general case programming practices (Horner, McDonnell, & Bellamy, 1986; Horner, Sprague, & Wilcox, 1982) to the problems presented by competing behaviors and ensures that the range of conditions under which the function of controlling stimuli should be changed is included in instructional examples. Although practical applications of the general case approach may involve instruction under different setting conditions (e.g., Horner, Jones, & Williams, 1985; Sprague & Horner, 1984), demonstrations and descriptions have focused primarily on systematic variations in specific task stimuli. It is suggested here that such an approach might profitably be extended to the more general stimulus context in which target behaviors are to be performed.

In cases where the competing behavior is associated with only one relevant stimulus (such as with a particular person or in a particular place), or with a very small number of relevant stimuli, instruction designed to change the function of controlling stimuli should involve the participation of the specific person or the presence of the particular stimulus event that seems to evoke the competing behavior. Marholin and Touchette (1979) have described this process as one in which controlling stimuli are "preprogrammed" (p. 317). If, however, the competing behavior is observed under a broad range of stimulus conditions, then general case logic should be applied not only to task characteristics but to the characteristics of the context in which the task is to be performed. Is a task, for example, to be performed at a variety of times during the day as in the case of dishwashing; should it be performed in a number of locations with different physical characteristics such as restaurants; will environmental elements within locations differ from time to time, as in situations that are sometimes, but not always, crowded or sometimes, but not always, noisy? The application of general case instruction to this problem of competing behaviors suggests that the teacher should identify those setting conditions in which the target behavior rather than the competing behavior should be displayed, and that teaching and test examples be chosen to sample variations in those conditions. In other words, if the target behavior must supplant the competing behavior in the morning and afternoon, in crowded and uncrowded areas where it is sometimes noisy and sometimes quiet, in the presence of familiar and unfamiliar persons, and so forth, then teaching and testing sites should include variations in those characteristics. The aim of this practice is to evoke and reinforce the new (efficient and reliable) behavior under the same *class* of stimulus conditions that had previously set the occasion for the competing behavior, and thereby change the function of those conditions (cf., Schroeder et al., 1984). In the absence of programming that adequately samples the range of setting variations that have previously controlled the competing behavior, it is possible that target behavior performance will be limited to an undesirable narrow range of stimulus conditions. Some new variation of conditions, then, might evoke the competing behavior rather than the target behavior (McDonnell et al., 1984; Ray, 1969).

Strategies within Nontraining Settings

On some occasions, a competing behavior within a student's repertoire may be so reliable and efficient that interventions applied in training situations will be insufficient to foster generalization. Grabbing, for example, will always permit access to desired items faster than requesting those items and waiting for someone to provide them. Teaching the student to be a more fluent pointer, then, might be an inadequate technique (when used alone) to produce sustained, generalized pointing (Horner & Budd, 1985). In such cases, it may be necessary to alter some component of those settings within which generalization is desired, as described in the paragraphs following.

Decrease the Efficiency and/or Reliability of Competing Behavior One possible alteration is to minimize the extent to which competing behaviors permit reliable and/or efficient access to reinforcers (Horner, 1971; Stolz & Wolf, 1969). This was the technique employed by Billingsley and Neel (1985) to promote the cross-setting use of "point" behavior.

The results in Figure 4 indicate the frequency of pointing and grabbing behaviors for a student during these conditions: baseline (when both grabbing and pointing were permitted) and deny (when grabbing was not allowed to produce food). The results indicate the value of reducing the efficiency of the competing behaviors.

Eliminate the Controlling Stimulus for Competing Behavior A second alteration, as suggested by Schroeder et al. (1984), is to eliminate the stimuli that evoke the competing behaviors from nontraining settings. Following this reasoning, if traffic noise seemed related to self-injurious behaviors (SIB) (which, in turn, interfered with the performance of community mobility skills), that noise might be effectively masked by music played

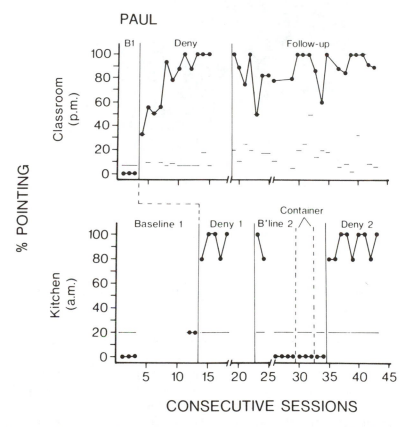

Figure 4. Percentage of pointing responses within acquisition (classroom) and generalization settings. (Reprinted with permission from Billingsley, F.F., & Neel, R.S. [1985]. Competing behaviors and their effects on skill generalization and maintenance. *Analysis and Intervention in Developmental Disabilities*, 5[4], 357–372.)

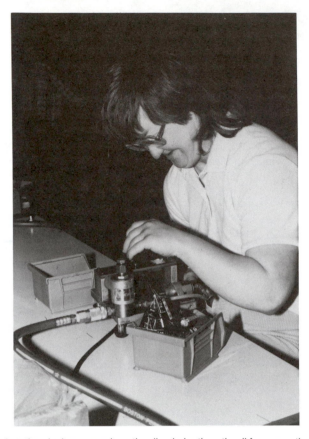

Efficient workstation design can reduce the discriminative stimuli for competing behaviors.

through the earphones of a personal stereo. If a specific toy, or class of toys, seemed to evoke stereotypical behaviors rather than appropriate play, those toys might be made unavailable to the individual. This approach is most practical where the stimuli controlling the competing behavior are irrelevant for the target skill.

The obvious drawback to the implementation of strategies in nontraining settings is that they require a "rearrangement of the natural environment" (Stokes & Baer, 1977, p. 354). In some situations in which generalization is required across a relatively narrow range of conditions, rearrangement may be relatively simple. Parents, for instance, could be trained not to assist their child in getting dressed in the morning *and* not to permit their child to engage in any other activity until he or she has completed independent dressing. Where generalization is expected across a broader range of situations and persons, however, the redesign of environments may be difficult to either implement or maintain.

IMPLICATIONS FOR RESEARCH

The implications of competing behaviors for generalization and maintenance in applied settings relate to both the methodology and content of future research.

Implications for Research Methodology

Identification of Existing Relationships   In research designed specifically to deal with the problems posed by competing behaviors, the behavioral functions of the competing stimulus control relationship should be documented prior to the implementation of the intervention. In the absence of such documentation, the effects of interventions could be misinterpreted and erroneous conclusions could result regarding the potential impact of response competition on skill performance. Recently, Carr and his colleagues conducted laboratory analogue analyses showing that undesirable behaviors served different functions for different students (cf., Carr, Chapter 10). The identification of the different functions permitted development of different treatments to reduce the excess behaviors. More work is needed on practical procedures for conducting functional analyses in applied settings, and then translating these analyses into effective interventions.

Assessment Methods   A major need currently exists to develop efficient and precise methods for assessing stimulus control relationships and the *strength* of those relationships in applied settings. Schroeder et al. (1984) suggested that "an important aspect of stimulus control research and, perhaps the most difficult aspect of conducting that research, is defining the functional stimulus. This difficulty stems from the multiplicity of stimuli that may come to control behavior, and the lack of correspondence that may occur between what the experimenter defines as a functional stimulus and what may actually control behavior" (p. 18). Similar sentiments have been expressed by others (e.g., Bijou & Baer, 1961; Liberty, 1986; Marholin & Touchette, 1979). In addition, much of the current theory is based on assumptions concerning the comparative strength of two competing stimulus control relationships. We need, therefore, to document not only whether a stimulus control relationship exists in applied settings but the magnitude of the relationship at a specified time as well. Work by Schreibman and her colleagues has addressed this need, and is reported in depth in Chapter 2.

The "Implications for Applied Settings" section of this chapter recommended a number of questions the practitioner might use to gain information related to particular competing behavior problems. Similar questions may also be of value to the researcher involved in intervention research dealing with generalization and maintenance; however, the extent to which answers to such questions will facilitate the systematic expansion and refinement of the existing knowledge base is likely to be limited in the absence of well-defined measurement systems and practices. Both direct observation in natural environments and analogue assessments are capable of providing important information. Observational methods for the purposes described, however, may be extremely time consuming, and analogue assessment situations may be difficult to design in many cases (Wolery & Billingsley, 1986). Assessment technology, therefore, is deserving of considerable research attention in the future.

Experimental Designs and Dependent Variables Although newly trained behaviors may supplant competing, excess behaviors under some conditions, the analysis presented herein and the research base to date indicate that obtained effects may be neither permanent nor observed in all situations. Experimental designs should permit the assessment of functional relationships between the acquisition, generalization, and maintenance of desirable target behaviors, and reductions in excess behaviors. This is more than a single, traditional design and the assessment of a single dependent variable can do (Hersen & Barlow, 1976; Kratochwill, 1978). Different designs employing multiple dependent variables will be needed across multiple studies. Billingsley and Neel (1985), for example, found it necessary to combine elements of three designs (multiple probe, multiple baseline across persons and settings, and withdrawal) in order to demonstrate functional relationships between the generalization and maintenance of a desired behavior (pointing for food) and the reduction of an undesired behavior (grabbing for food). Horner, Albin, and Mank (1986) employed an extended within-subject replication design in which levels of both competing and target behaviors were assessed in training and nontraining settings to investigate the effects of prior learning on a newly acquired stimulus control relationship. As the relationships under investigation become increasingly complex, it is reasonable to anticipate that the measurement of more than one dependent variable will be required and that design elements will need frequently to be arranged in unfamiliar (and flexible) combinations.

Implications for Research Content

Identification of the Functions of Behaviors In order to deal effectively with competing behavior problems, the functions served by those behaviors require documentation. As noted by Carr and Durand (1985a) and Iwata, Dorsey, Slifer, Bauman, and Richman (1982), aggression/disruption and self-injurious behaviors can serve several functions such as sensory stimulation, producing attention from others, and escaping from undesirable situations. This work has provided a model for the systematic investigation of behavioral functions. Many additional examples are required, however, that focus on a broader range of both behaviors (which may be more subtle than aggression or SIB) and specific functions.

Predictive Validity of the Analysis   The analysis presented in this chapter (Figures 2 and 3) suggests that certain approaches are likely to be more successful than others. The predictive validity of the analysis, therefore, needs to be determined. For example, in most cases it seems improbable that an approach that focused solely on increasing the fluency of the target behavior would improve generalization or maintenance within situations where the competing behavior and the target behavior result in entirely different reinforcers. Such an approach, however, might frequently be effective when the target response and competing response achieve the *same* reinforcer. The relationships presented in Figure 2 should also contribute to a functional analysis for intervening on excess behaviors that could augment currently recommended intervention hierarchies (Evans & Meyer, 1985). By way of illustration, if David bites himself when presented with tasks/demands, a stimulus control analysis would suggest that intervention should differ if: 1) biting is controlled by the presentation of tasks/demands (competing behavior under control of stimuli within the instructional universe), versus 2) biting only occurs when his sister is present (competing behavior under control of specific irrelevant stimulus, versus 3) biting only occurs when he is in large, crowded areas such as department stores (competing behavior under control of broad, nonmanipulatable, irrelevant stimuli).

Breaking versus Suppressing Stimulus Control   Of particular concern for both theoretical and applied researchers is the possible difference in the generalization and maintenance of new skills that might be observed when the stimulus control for competing behaviors is broken, as opposed to when that stimulus control is suppressed. Where an intervention is implemented specifically to suppress competing behavior in training settings, the literature strongly suggests that the behavior may come under the control of stimuli associated with the intervention and that the competing behavior may reappear when those stimuli are not present (cf., Neel, 1978). It would, therefore, be productive to investigate whether methods designed to break old stimulus control relationships and replace them with new ones (e.g., increasing the relative efficiency/reliability of target behaviors) would produce more reliable and enduring performance in nontraining settings than methods that involve the suppression of relationships.

Even more basic, of course, is the need to establish with greater precision those conditions that are necessary and sufficient to actually break an existing relationship. Schroeder et al. (1984) have noted that "until those conditions which abolish versus those which reduce the frequency of a relation are delineated, it will be impossible to know if procedures that change the function of the controlling stimulus will abolish the previous relation or merely suppress its frequency for a period of time" (p. 20).

Teaching Response Classes   Finally, the extent to which new behaviors that are taught as response classes are likely to be more durable and shielded from competing behaviors than behaviors that are taught as individual responses should be investigated. If only a single (desirable) response form is available to an individual, and that form fails to achieve the reinforcing function owing to changing environmental conditions, it is possible that the individual may then exhibit the competing (undesirable) behavior in order to accomplish the function. On the other hand, if a variety of desirable response forms are taught that produce the same effect, the individual will have alternatives to the competing behavior in his or her repertoire, should a particular desirable form fail to attain the reinforcing function. The instruction of appropriate response classes, then, could provide students with the means to adjust responses to variations in environmental demands without employing undesirable competing behaviors.

SUMMARY

A comprehensive technology of behavior must include analysis of the mechanisms by which stimulus control relationships compete in applied settings. This chapter presents one approach for examining competing behavior. The major messages from this approach are: 1) human behavior in applied settings is more complex than a simple $S \rightarrow R \rightarrow S$ model can describe; 2) procedures are needed that allow adequate assessment of both target and competing behaviors prior to the construction of interventions; and 3) effective interventions should include manipulation of three variables: antecedent events, the efficiency and/ or reliability of target responses, *and* consequences for both target and competing behaviors. Although it adds complexity to study of the problem, the competing behavior analysis extends our notion of behavior management from an emphasis on obtaining transient change to an emphasis on durable behavior modification that results in meaningful life-style changes.

REFERENCES

Albin, R.W., McDonell, J.J., & Wilcox, B. (1987). Designing interventions to meet activity goals. In B. Wilcox & G.T. Bellamy, *A comprehensive guide to* The Activities Catalogue: *An alternative curriculum for youth and adults with severe disabilities* (pp. 63–88). Baltimore: Paul H. Brookes Publishing Co.

Bandura, A. (1969). *Principles of behavior modification*. New York: Holt, Rinehart, and Winston.

Becker, W., Engelmann, S., & Thomas, D. (1975). *Teaching 2: Cognitive learning and instruction* (pp. 57–92). Chicago: Science Research Associates.

Bijou, S.W., & Baer, D.M. (1961). *Child development I: A systematic and empirical theory*. New York: Appleton-Century-Crofts.

Billingsley, F.F., (1984). Where are the generalized outcomes? (An examination of instructional objectives). *Journal of The Association for Persons with Severe Handicaps, 9*(3), 186–192.

Billingsley, F.F., & Neel, R.S. (1985). Competing behaviors and their effects on skill generalization and maintenance. *Analysis and Intervention in Developmental Disabilities, 5*, 357–372.

Brown, L., Branston, M.B., Hamre-Nietupski, S., Pumpian, J., Certo, N., & Gruenwald, L. (1979). A strategy for developing chronological age appropriate and functional curricular content for severely handicapped adolescents and young adults. *Journal of Special Education, 13*, 81–90.

Cahoon, D.D. (1968). Symptom substitution and behavior therapies: A reappraisal. *Psychological Bulletin, 69*, 149–158.

Carr, E.G., & Durand, V.M. (1985a). Reducing behavior problems through functional communication training. *Journal of Applied Behavior Analysis, 18*, 111–126.

Carr, E.G., & Durand, V.M. (1985b). The social-communicative basis of severe behavior problems in children. In S. Reiss & R. Bootzin (Eds.), *Theoretical issues in behavior therapy* (pp. 219–254). New York: Academic Press.

Carr, E.G., & Kologinsky, E. (1983). Acquisition of sign language by autistic children II: Spontaneity and generalization effects. *Journal of Applied Behavior Analysis, 16*, 297–314.

Eason, L.J., White, M., & Newsom, C. (1982). Generalized reduction of self-stimulatory behavior: An effect of teaching appropriate play to autistic children. *Analysis and Intervention in Developmental Disabilities, 2*, 157–169.

Engelmann, S., & Carnine, D. (1982). *Theory of instruction: Principles and applications* (pp. 1–54). New York: Irvington.

Engelmann, S., & Colvin, G. (1983). *Generalized compliance training: A direct-instruction program for managing severe behavior problems*. Austin, TX: PRO-ED.

Evans, I.M., & Meyer, L.H. (1985). *An educative approach to behavior problems: A practical decision model for interventions with severely handicapped learners*. Baltimore: Paul H. Brookes Publishing Co.

Falvey, M.A. (1986). *Community-based curriculum: Instructional strategies for students with severe handicaps*. Baltimore: Paul H. Brookes Publishing Co.

Favell, J.E., McGimsey, J.F., & Schell, R.M. (1982). Treatment of self-injury by providing alternate sensory activities. *Analysis and Intervention in Developmental Disabilities, 2*, 83–104.

Hersen, M., & Barlow, D. (1976). *Single case experimental designs: Strategies for studying behavior change* (pp. 198–222). New York: Pergamon.

Honig, W.K., & Urcuioli, P.J. (1981). The legacy of Guttman and Kalish (1956): 25 years of research on stimulus generalization. *Journal of Experimental Analysis of Behavior, 36*(3), 405–445.

Horner, R.D. (1971). Establishing the use of crutches by a mentally retarded spina bifida child. *Journal of Applied Behavior Analysis, 4*, 183–189.

Horner, R.H., Albin, R.W., & Mank, D.M. (1986). *Effects of prior learning on the generalized suppression of inappropriate verbalizations: A case study.* Manuscript submitted for publication.

Horner, R.H., Albin, R.W., & Ralph, G. (1986). Generalization with precision: The role of negative teaching examples in the instruction of generalized grocery item selection. *Journal of The Association for Persons with Severe Handicaps, 11*(4), 300–308.

Horner, R.H., Bellamy, G.T., & Colvin, G.T. (1984). Responding in the presence of nontrained stimuli: Implications of generalization error patterns. *Journal of The Association for Persons with Severe Handicaps, 9,* 287–296.

Horner, R.H., & Budd, C.M. (1985). Teaching manual sign language to a nonverbal student: Generalization of sign use and collateral reduction of maladaptive behavior. *Education and Training of the Mentally Retarded, 20*(1), 39–47.

Horner, R.H., Jones, D., & Williams, J.A. (1985). Teaching generalized street crossing to individuals with moderate and severe mental retardation. *Journal of The Association for Persons with Severe Handicaps, 10,* 71–78.

Horner, R.H., McDonnell, J.J., & Bellamy, G.T. (1986). Teaching generalized skills: General case instruction in simulation and community settings. In R.H. Horner, L.H. Meyer, & H.D. Fredericks (Eds.), *Education of learners with severe handicaps: Exemplary service strategies* (pp. 289–314). Baltimore: Paul H. Brookes Publishing Co.

Horner, R.H., Sprague, J., & Wilcox, B. (1982). General case programming for community activities. In B. Wilcox & G.T. Bellamy, *Design of high school programs for severely handicapped students* (pp. 61–98). Baltimore: Paul H. Brookes Publishing Co.

Horner, R.H., Williams, J.A., & Stevely, J.D. (1987). Acquisition of generalized telephone use by students with severe mental retardation. *Research in Developmental Disabilities, 8,* 229–247.

Iwata, B.A., Dorsey, M.F., Slifer, K.J., Bauman, K.E., & Richman, G.S. (1982). Toward a functional analysis of self-injury. *Analysis and Intervention in Developmental Disabilities, 2,* 3–20.

Kamin, L.J. (1968). Attention-like processes in classical conditioning. In M.R. Jones (Ed.), *Miami symposium on the prediction of behavior, 1967: Aversive stimulation.* Miami: University of Miami Press.

Kazdin, A.E. (1980). *Behavior modification in applied settings* (2nd ed.). Homewood, IL: Dorsey Press.

Kratochwill, T.R. (1978). Foundations of time-series research. In T.R. Kratochwill (Ed.), *Single subject research: Strategies for evaluating change* (pp. 1–100). New York: Academic Press.

Leighand, S. (1984). On "setting events" and related concepts. *Behavior Analyst, 7*(1), 41–46.

Liberty, K.A. (1986, May). *Analysis of stimulus effects on response rates.* Paper presented at the Twelfth Annual Association for Behavior Analysis Convention, Milwaukee.

Liberty, K.A., & Billingsley, F.F. (1985). *Strategies for generalization.* Unpublished manuscript, University of Washington, Washington Research Organization, Seattle.

Mackintosh, J.H. (1977). Stimulus control: Attentional factors. In W.K. Honig & J.E.R. Staddon (Eds.), *Handbook of operant behavior* (pp. 481–513). New Jersey: Prentice-Hall.

Marholin, D., II, & Touchette, P.E. (1979). The role of stimulus control and response consequences. In A. Goldstein & F. Kanfer (Eds.), *Maximizing treatment gains* (pp. 303–351). New York: Academic Press.

McDonnell, J.J., & Horner, R.H. (1985). Effects of in vivo and simulation-plus-in vivo training on the acquisition and generalization of a grocery item search strategy by high school students with severe handicaps. *Analysis and Intervention in Developmental Disabilities, 5,* 323–344.

McDonnell, J.J., Horner, R.H., & Williams, J.A. (1984). Comparison of three strategies for teaching generalized grocery purchasing to high school students with severe handicaps. *Journal of The Association for Persons with Severe Handicaps, 9,* 123–133.

Michael, J.L. (1983). Distinguishing between discriminative and motivational functions of stimulus. *Journal of the Experimental Analysis of Behavior, 37,* 149–155.

Neel, R.S. (1978). Research findings regarding the use of punishment procedures with severely behavior disordered children. In. F.H. Wood & K.C. Lakin (Eds.), *Punishment and aversive stimulation in special education: Legal, theoretical, and practical issues in their use with emotionally disturbed children and youth* (pp. 65–83). Minneapolis: Department of Psychoeducational Studies, University of Minnesota.

Newman, F.L., & Baron, M.R. (1965). Stimulus generalization along the dimension of angularity. *Journal of Comparative and Physiological Psychology, 60,* 59–63.

O'Brien, F., Azrin, N.H., & Bugle, C. (1972). Training profoundly retarded children to stop crawling. *Journal of Applied Behavior Analysis, 5,* 131–137.

Ray, B.A. (1969). Selective attention: The effects of combining stimuli which control incompatible behavior. *Journal of the Experimental Analysis of Behavior, 12,* 539–550.

Rudolph, R.L., Honig, W.K., & Gerry, J.E. (1969). Effects of monochromatic rearing on the acquisition of stimulus control. *Journal of Comparative and Physiological Psychology, 67,* 50–57.

Schroeder, S.R., Bickel, W.K., & Richmond, G. (1984, October). *Primary and secondary prevention of self-injurious behaviors: A life-long problem.* Paper presented at Self-Injurious Behavior Symposium, Kansas City, KS.

Solomon, R.W., & Wahler, R.G. (1973). Peer reinforcement control of classroom problem behavior. *Journal of Applied Behavior Analysis, 6,* 49–56.

Sprague, J.R., & Horner, R.H. (1984). The effects of single instance, multiple instance, and general case training on generalized vending machine use by moderately and severely handicapped students. *Journal of Applied Behavior Analysis, 17,* 273–278.

Staddon, J.E.R. (1977). Schedule-induced behavior. In W.K. Honig & J.E.R. Staddon (Eds.), *Handbook of operant behavior* (pp. 125–152). Englewood Cliffs, NJ: Prentice-Hall.

Stokes, T.F., & Baer, D.M. (1977). An implicit technology of generalization. *Journal of Applied Behavior Analysis, 10,* 349–367.

Stolz, S.B., & Wolf, M.M. (1969). Visually discriminated behavior in a "blind" adolescent retardate. *Journal of Applied Behavior Analysis, 2,* 65–77.

Terrace, H. (1966). Stimulus control. In W. Honig (Ed.), *Operation behavior areas of research and application* (pp. 271–344). New York: Appleton-Century-Crofts.

Wahler, R.G., & Fox, J.J. (1981). Setting events in applied behavior analysis: Toward a conceptual and methodological expansion. *Journal of Applied Behavior Analysis, 14* (327–338).

White, O.R. (1985). Aim star wars (setting aims that compete), Episodes II and III.

Journal of Precision Teaching, 5, 86–94.

Wilcox, B., & Bellamy, G.T. (1982). *Design of high school programs for severely handicapped students.* Baltimore: Paul H. Brookes Publishing Co.

Wolery, M., & Billingsley, F.F. (1986). *Form, function, and functional behavior: Clarification of terms.* Manuscript submitted for publication.

Wolery, M., & Gast, D.L. (1984). Effective and efficient procedures for the transfer of stimulus control. *Topics in Early Childhood Special Education, 4*(3), 52–77.

Chapter 10

Functional Equivalence as a Mechanism of Response Generalization

Edward G. Carr

The search to discover a psychological process capable of producing broad treatment gains has long preoccupied clinicians and educators. Seldom do we wish to change only a single behavior. Instead, we hope that by intervening on one class of behaviors, other classes of behavior that have not been the target of intervention will also change in a desirable direction. This phenomenon has been referred to as response generalization (Bandura, 1969).

It is interesting that many nonbehavioral therapies operate on the assumption that response generalization will occur if therapy is carried out competently. For example, consider the use of psychoanalytic therapy for an aggressive adolescent. The psychoanalyst would not typically intervene on the aggression per se. Instead, effort would be expended to help the adolescent gain insight into underlying intrapsychic conflicts. Thus, during the course of treatment, a young man might learn that his aggression is a function of unconscious anger directed at his parents. The theory is that once the individual acquires this insight, aggressive behavior will disappear even though there was no direct attempt to ameliorate it. The change in aggression would constitute a true example of response generalization. By intervening on one class of behaviors (insight), the psychoanalyst causes changes in other classes of behavior (aggression) that have not been the target of intervention.

Behaviorists, of course, have been critical of psychoanalysis on both theoretical and empirical grounds. However, it remains true that unlike psychoanalysts, behaviorists have been slow in pursuing response generalization as the major goal of treatment, and even slower in developing a theory to account for the phenomenon. The intent of this chapter is to begin to develop a behavioral theory of response generalization. The central thesis presented is that functional equivalence is an important mechanism mediating response generalization.

Definition of Terms

Response Class   A *response class* is defined as a group of two or more topographically different behaviors, all of which have the same effect on the environment. Typically, the common effect involves producing a specific class of reinforcers. In this sense, the definition of response class is indistinguishable from the definition of the operant.

Response Generalization   This author defines *response generalization* as the change that occurs in one class of responses (R_1) when another class of responses (R_2) is manipulated. The change in R_1 occurs in spite of the fact that R_1 is not directly manipulated. Historically, the term *response generalization* has been restricted to the situation in which R_1 and R_2 both increase. This chapter's position is that the direction in which R_1 and R_2 change is not as important as the reasons for the change. Thus, there is no purpose in describing the various types of change using distinct labels such as positive and negative side effects, positive and negative covariation, or a variety of other terms that appear in the literature. The term, *response generalization,* is arguably the best one to use because it preserves the fundamental notion of generalization as a spread-of-effects phenomenon (Mostofsky, 1965). In stimulus generalization, for example, there is a spread of effects from the original learning situation to new situations. In a parallel manner, response generalization connotes a spread of effects from the original response target to other responses. The clinical examples described in this chapter all involve response generalization phenomena in which an undesirable response class (R_1) decreases when a desirable response class (R_2) increases following intervention.

Functional Equivalence   Functional equivalence is said to occur when two (or more) response classes are maintained by the same reinforcer class. For example, reaching for a cookie and saying the word *cookie* are both maintained by the reinforcer class represented by cookies. In addition, all possible motoric variations of the reaching behavior constitute one response class, and all possible vocal variations of the spoken word *cookie* constitute a second response class. Yet, in spite of the fact that the two response classes are quite distinct *topographically,* they are nonetheless considered to be identical from a *functional* perspective because both sets of behaviors are maintained by the same class of reinforcers, namely, cookies.

The task of the research scientist is to determine what function each of the response classes of interest serves; that is, what classes of reinforcers are involved. Then, the task becomes one of empirically establishing an equivalence between the response classes so as to enhance response generalization. This strategy is the central focus of this chapter and is illustrated in the pages that follow by means of four clinical examples involving autistic leading, severe behavior problems, stereotypy, and echolalia.

AUTISTIC LEADING

Autistic children, particularly those who are nonverbal, often engage in a behavior referred to as leading (Kanner, 1943). For example, a child who wishes to go outside may lead an adult by the hand over to a door. The child will then place the adult's hand on the doorknob and wait. Often, this behavior is viewed as primitive and undesirable. Therefore, it is ignored or, at best, responded to irregularly in the hope that it will disappear and be replaced with a more sophisticated response. This author has attempted to deal with the problem more systematically.

The first step is to determine what function autistic leading serves. One way of accomplishing this goal is to set up an analog situation resembling that encountered in the daily life of the child. In line with this strategy, this author and colleagues carried out a functional analysis of autistic leading in four preschool children who displayed a number of autistic features (Kemp & Carr, 1986). Each child was initially observed to lead his classroom teacher by the hand whenever the teacher placed desired objects out of reach. The child would typically raise the teacher's hand toward the inaccessible object. The author duplicated this situation in the laboratory so as to make a more formal assessment. Specifically, a child was allowed to play with a preferred toy for a short period of time. Then the toy was removed and placed high on a shelf out of reach. Each child engaged in autistic leading when confronted with this situation, and reliably terminated the behavior when the adult returned the toy to the child. The analysis clearly indicated that "preferred toy out of reach" was an antecedent controlling variable for autistic leading. This obervation made it plausible to infer that leading served a request function for the chld. That is, it was functionally equivalent to saying "I want the toy." However, since the children did not speak, autistic leading could be viewed as a prevocal form of communication.

Interestingly, young normal children also display prevocal communication. Therefore, the literature on these children may provide a framework for selecting replacement behaviors for autistic leading. The evidence suggests that during the first 2 years of life, children use a variety of prevocal behaviors communicatively. These behaviors include reaching, grabbing, directed looking, and even leading (Bates, Camaioni, & Volterra, 1975; Wellman & Lempers, 1977). Over the same period of time, the frequency of pointing gradually increases and supplants these other behaviors (Leung & Rheingold, 1981; Wellman & Lempers, 1977). Pointing is established as a prominent form of communication by age 2 (Leung & Rheingold, 1981; Murphy, 1978). The literature on normal child development thus suggests that pointing and leading can both serve a request function, and that pointing is developmentally more advanced. These facts imply that functional equivalence exists between leading and pointing. Therefore, strengthening the latter should weaken the former. This relationship is depicted in the first row of Table 1.

Will functional equivalence result in response generalization as predicted? This author and colleagues tested this possibility with the four children mentioned previously. Again, each child was permitted to play for a short period of time with a preferred toy, and then the toy was placed out of reach. Before the child could engage in autistic leading, however, he was physically prompted to point to the toy. When he pointed, he was given the toy once again. This procedure was repeated a number of times, during which the prompt was slowly faded. At no time during training did the child experience extinction trials for leading. In spite of the absence of any direct contingency on leading, that behavior permanently decreased to negligible levels once pointing was firmly established. This outcome therefore constitutes an example of response generalization plausibly mediated through the functional equivalence of leading and pointing.

Table 1. Four pairs of response classes that are functionally equivalent and the nature of that equivalence

Response class 1	Response class 2	Common function
Autistic leading	Prevocal communication (pointing)	Request for object
Aggression/self-injury/ tantrums	Speech: "Help me." _or_ Speech: "Am I doing good work?"	Escape from aversive stimulus _or_ Request for attention
Stereotypy	Speech: "Help me."	Escape from aversive stimulus
Echolalia	Speech: "I don't know."	Escape from aversive stimulus (expresses lack of comprehension)

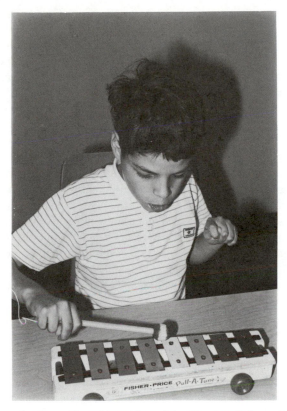

Response generalization can be achieved through functional equivalence. The toy was obtained by pointing instead of leading the teacher to the toy.

SEVERE BEHAVIOR PROBLEMS

A situation commonly seen with some autistic children is that they will scream and tantrum when they have to go to the bathroom. If a teacher were to follow textbook treatment advice rigidly, then a DRO (differential reinforcement of other behavior) procedure would be tried as a means of controlling the tantrums. Paradoxically, such a procedure might consist of giving the child a small quantity of juice for every minute that the child was quiet. This strategy is clearly inappropriate since it would exacerbate the toileting problem. For that reason, experienced teachers would not implement the procedure described. Yet, on purely technical grounds, DRO is often appropriate. In the instance given, however, it lacks face validity. The feeling that the procedure lacks validity stems from an intuitive notion, shared by many people, that screaming may represent a primitive attempt at communication (Carr & Durand, 1987). Therefore, a more appropriate treatment strategy would consist of teaching the child to ask to go to the bathroom. Can we improve on these intuitive notions by subjecting them to systematic empirical analysis? This author believes that the answer is yes and, further, that it relates to the issue of response generalization.

Consider first the literature on normal children. Data exist showing that 3-year-olds who have poor expressive language skills are much more likely to display a variety of behavior problems than same-age peers who have good expressive skills (Stevenson & Richman, 1978). Related to these findings is a growing body of evidence that behaviors such as crying and aggression may indeed serve communicative functions in children who have immature language development. For example, in a longitudinal study of infant crying during the first year of life, Bell and Ainsworth (1972) found that crying became increasingly socially oriented as the infant grew older. Eventually, crying was most likely to occur when children were in close proximity to their mothers. Further, crying evoked specific maternal responses such as picking up and holding the child, followed (in order of probability), by vocalizing and interacting, feeding, approaching and touching, and offering toys. Infant crying functioned as a protoimperative (Bates et al., 1975), that is, a preverbal form of requesting. A similar point was made by Brownlee and Bakeman (1981) in a study of aggression in toddlers. These investigators found that certain forms of aggressive behavior (open-handed hitting) exhibited by a child had the effect of driving other children away. The finding was interpreted to mean that aggression could serve as a nonverbal protest behavior that communicated the notion, "Leave me alone." Other forms of aggressive behavior (hitting a second child softly with a stuffed animal) had the effect of promoting pleasant social interaction. Brownlee and Bakeman speculated that these behaviors functioned as nonverbal requests for attention; that is, they expressed the notion, "Hey, wanna play?"

The speculations made in the two studies reviewed imply that if children were to develop more sophisticated (effective) means of protest and of getting attention, then these same children would give up many of their immature behaviors. In fact, it is commonly observed that children often "grow out of" their infantile behavior patterns. The two studies cited provide data that may bear on the reason why positive changes occur. In particular, both studies found that as gestural and verbal communicative abilities improved, crying and aggression decreased markedly. These findings imply that behavior problems and communication can be functionally related in normal children. Is the same true for developmentally disabled children?

Two studies suggest that behavior problems and communication skill are indeed linked in the developmentally disabled. The first study (Shodell & Reiter, 1968) was based on a sample of 58 autistic children. Parents and teachers of the children were asked to fill out questionnaires designed to measure the frequency of self-injury over a 10-day period. Categories of self-injury included head-banging, self-biting, and self-scratching. The major finding was that 47% of those who had poor communication skills were self-injurious, but only 19% of those who had good communication skills were. In the second study (Talkington, Hall, & Altman, 1971), a sample of 70 noncommunicating retarded persons was compared with a sample of 70 communicating retarded persons. The individuals, who were institutionalized, were rated by ward personnel on various categories of aggression such as "breaks windows," "requires restraint," and "destroys property." On these categories, the noncommunicators were rated as significantly more aggressive than the communicators. Based on the evidence presented, it appears that the inverse relationship between behavior problems and communication skill seen in normal children is also seen in developmentally disabled children.

The studies reviewed, although suggestive, are correlational in nature. To further our understanding of the issues involved, it is necessary to carry out additional research. First, one would have to perform a functional analysis of the behavior problems. Second, based on this analysis, one would select specific communicative alternatives to the behavior problems and test the efficacy of these alternatives.

Consider first the functional analysis of behavior problems. An extensive literature exists suggesting that the factors responsible for the maintenance of socially motivated behavior problems fall into two broad classes: escape behavior, controlled by negative reinforcement processes, and attention-seeking behavior, controlled by positive reinforcement processes (Carr & Durand, 1985a). Escape behavior typically becomes worse in response to aversive stimuli. For example, when a child is repeatedly presented with a difficult academic task (presumably an aversive stimulus), one often observes increases in a variety of behavior problems such as aggression (Carr, Newsom, & Binkoff, 1980), self-injury (Carr, 1977; Carr, Newsom, & Binkoff, 1976), and tantrums (Carr & Newsom, 1985). These same problems decline to low levels when easy task demands are presented. In contrast, attention-seeking behavior problems are generally not affected by task difficulty per se. Instead, the degree to which attention is presented contingently on the display of behavior problems is a major determinant of the frequency with which such problems occur. Contingent attention has been shown to increase the rate of self-injurious behavior (Carr & McDowell, 1980; Lovaas, Freitag, Gold, & Kassorla, 1965), aggression (Brown & Elliott, 1965; Wahler, 1967), and tantrums (Williams, 1959). Another way of viewing these data is to note that low levels of adult attention often provoke behavior problems. These problems, once displayed, cause adults to increase their attention to the children.

The literature cited suggests that a decrease in the level of adult attention should function as a discriminative stimulus for behavior problems in attention-seeking children. Likewise, the shift from easy to difficult demands should evoke behavior problems in children who are escape motivated with respect to instructional situations. These considerations have allowed this author and V.M. Durand to develop assessment procedures to aid in the functional analysis of classroom behavior problems (Carr & Durand, 1985b).

First, in order to assess for escape-motivated problems, Carr and Durand (1985b) confronted developmentally disabled children with two sets of tasks. One set was preselected to generate only 25% correct responding (difficult task); the other was preselected to generate 100% correct responding (easy task). Second, in order to assess for attention-motivated problems, the level of adult attention was manipulated so as to produce high and low levels. In the high-attention condition, the adult spent 100% of the instructional session interacting with the child. In the low-attention condition, the adult spent most of the session teaching other children, with the result that the target child was attended to only 33% of the time. The results of this functional analysis were as follows. Some children became disruptive when the adult shifted from easy to difficult tasks. These individuals were labeled as escape motivated. Some children became disruptive when the adult shifted from high to low levels of attention. These individuals were labeled as attention seeking. Finally, a few children showed both the escape and attention-seeking patterns.

Following a functional analysis, it becomes possible to select replacements for the problem behaviors. The literature on both normal and developmentally disabled children implies that if communicative behaviors are judiciously selected and strengthened, there may be a concomitant decrease in problem behaviors. This outcome would not only be clinically desirable but also would be relevant to furthering our understanding of the nature of response generalization.

One could predict that teaching children communicative alternatives that serve the same social function as the behavior problems would produce a decrease in the level of those problems. In contrast, teaching alternatives that serve nonequivalent functions would not. Figure 1 presents data on four children who were involved in a test of this hypothesis (Carr & Durand, 1985b). The labels "Difficult 100" and "Easy 33" refer to combinations of control conditions, the details of which are peripheral to the present discussion. The important point is that the label "Difficult 100" identifies three of the children as being escape motivated, and the label "Easy 33" identifies two of the children as being attention seeking. What communicative alternatives can be chosen that serve the same social function as the behavior problems? Escape-motivated problems could plausibly be dealt with by teaching the child to request help ("Help me") when confronted with a difficult task. This request should elicit

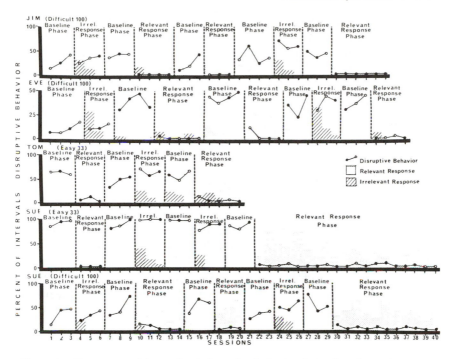

Figure 1. Percentage of intervals of disruptive behavior during baseline, relevant response, and irrelevant response phases. The level of relevant verbal responses is indicated by stippled bars and that of irrelevant verbal responses by hatched bars. (Reprinted with permission from Carr, E.G., & Durand, V.M. [1985b]. Reducing behavior problems through functional communication training. *Journal of Applied Behavior Analysis, 18, 122.* Copyright 1985 by the Society for the Experimental Analysis of Behavior.)

teacher assistance, thereby decreasing task difficulty and avoiding failure. In a real sense, the child can be said to have escaped from the aversive task, albeit in a socially appropriate and desirable manner, namely, by talking. Attention-seeking behavior could plausibly be dealt with by instructing the child on how to solicit teacher attention through verbal means. For example, the child could show completed desk work to the teacher and ask, "Am I doing good work?" This behavior should produce teacher attention in situations in which such attention would otherwise not be forthcoming. In this manner, the child is able to deal with low levels of teacher attention without having to resort to severe behavior problems. Figure 1 refers to the two verbal responses just described as "Relevant Response," denoting the idea that each response is relevant to the motivation of the behavior problem that it seeks to replace. That is, escape phrases are relevant to dealing with aversive tasks, and attention phrases are relevant to dealing with low levels of adult attention. If one were to teach an escape phrase for a situation in which a low level of adult attention was the critical variable, or an attention phrase for dealing with a situation in which task difficulty was important, then one would be teaching irrelevant phrases. This condition was made part of the experiment, to rule out the possibility that merely training children to utter *any* verbal phrase would be effective. The control condition just described is labeled in Figure 1 as "Irrelevant Response." As can be seen from the figure, teaching irrelevant responses did not result in systematic decreases in behavior problems. In fact, the level of behavior problems was no different than that obtained in a baseline condition in which no verbal responses were taught. However, when relevant responses were taught and appropriately consequated by the adult, behavior problems decreased to negligible levels. Interestingly, similar data have been produced when sign language is taught as an alternative to behavior problems (Horner & Budd, 1985). Thus, the mode of communication is less important than the consequences involved.

To understand the significance of the data just discussed, one must realize that at no point was any contingency applied to the problem behaviors. Yet, in spite of this fact, problems declined as communicative responses were strengthened. This outcome constitutes another example of response generalization. Importantly, when phrases were taught that were functionally equivalent to the behavior problems (relevant responses), response generalization was observed (i.e., the problems decreased). This relationship is summarized in the second row of Table 1. In contrast, when functionally nonequivalent phrases were taught (irrelevant responses), response generalization was not observed. These data serve to illustrate the point that, in the circumstances described, response generalization can be expected to occur only when functional equivalence between response classes has been carefully programmed.

STEREOTYPY

Autistic children frequently engage in a variety of stereotyped motor acts such as rocking, hand-flapping, and spinning objects. Many researchers have speculated that such behaviors are self-stimulatory in nature and are maintained by the sensory consequences they produce (Baumeister & Forehand, 1972; Berkson & Davenport, 1962). Recent evidence supports this viewpoint (Rincover, Cook, Peoples, & Packard, 1979; Wolery, Kirk, & Gast, 1985). For example, Rincover et al. (1979) demonstrated that the repetitive plate-spinning behavior of one autistic boy was maintained by its auditory consequences. When the sound that the plate made on a hard surface was eliminated by carpeting that surface, the stereotyped spinning behavior was dramatically reduced.

The literature suggests that sensory consequences may not be the only factor controlling stereotypy. A number of studies provide evidence that repeti-

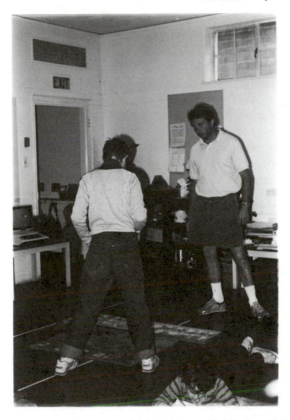

Functionally equivalent phrases can result in response generalization. This student's disruptive, attention-getting behavior decreased when he was taught an appropriate way to ask for teacher attention.

tive motor behavior sometimes increases when an individual is frustrated (Baumeister & Forehand, 1973). In one study (Forehand & Baumeister, 1971), four individuals with retardation were prevented from obtaining reinforcers to which they previously had access. Blocking of a goal response constitutes a frustration procedure. Significantly, this frustration procedure produced an increase in body-rocking. Data such as these imply that stereotyped behavior may at times be influenced by operant factors. This notion finds strong support in studies demonstrating that different schedules of reinforcement produce different rates of stereotyped acts (Baumeister & Forehand, 1973). Durand and Carr (1987) followed up on the conditioning theory of stereotypy by creating a situation in which another operant factor, negative reinforcement, could be studied.

Four children who were autistic or who displayed a variety of autistic features were involved. Classroom observation of these children suggested a correlation between task difficulty and the level of body-rocking and hand-flapping. Therefore, Durand and Carr (1987) performed a functional analysis to determine whether escape factors were involved. Two pieces of evidence suggested that the stereotyped behaviors were indeed escape motivated. First, stereotypy became more frequent when task difficulty increased. Second, when timeout was made contingent on stereotypy, the stereotyped behavior again increased in frequency. Timeout involves a cessation of demands. It is important to note, therefore, that when stereotypy results in the removal of demands, the stereotyped behavior increases. This finding makes sense only when one views demands as an aversive stimulus. In that case, stereotyped behavior is an escape response maintained by the negative reinforcement represented by the removal of demands.

If the function of stereotypy is to terminate aversive stimuli, then one would predict that providing children with other behaviors that serve the same function should result in a decrease in the level of stereotyped behavior. As was the case with severe behavior problems (described earlier), Durand and Carr (1987) chose to teach the child to request help ("Help me") when confronted with difficult task demands. In this way, the child could receive assistance from the teacher, who would simplify the task by prompting the correct answer. This response therefore removed the aversive stimulus (difficult demands) and was functionally equivalent to the stereotyped behavior. The relationship between the two response classes is summarized in the third row of Table 1. Figure 2 shows the results of the manipulation. Prior to training, each child showed high levels of body-rocking or hand-flapping.

After a communicative response was taught, that response increased in frequency (shaded histograms in Figure 2). Most importantly, stereotyped behavior decreased following the communication intervention. Since the stereotypy was not subjected to any intervention, the fact that it decreased constitutes another instance of response generalization. Again, it was shown that functional equivalence can be a key variable in mediating response generalization.

ECHOLALIA

Half of all autistic children are echolalic (Rutter, 1966), and this speech characteristic is one of the diagnostic features of autism. Although echolalia can occur either immediately or after a delay following what another person has said, most research has focused on immediate echolalia, and it is this phenomenon that is discussed here.

Immediate echolalia involves the direct parroting of what another person has just said. For example, an adult may approach a child and ask "Where do

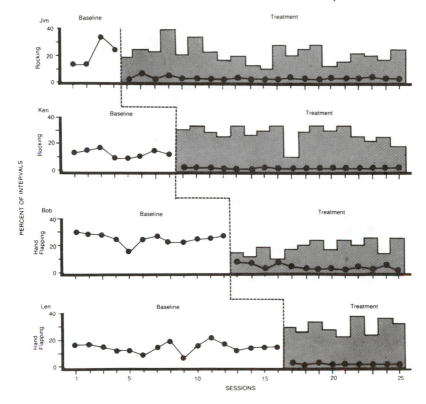

Figure 2. Percentage of intervals of stereotyped behavior during baseline and following communication training. The shaded areas represent the rate of subjects' use of the phrase "Help me." (Reprinted with permission from Durand, V.M., & Carr, E.G. [1987]. Social influences on "self-stimulatory" behavior: Analysis and treatment application. *Journal of Applied Behavior Analysis, 20,* 119–132. Copyright 1987 by the Society for the Experimental Analysis of Behavior.)

you live?" to which the child responds, "Where do you live?" What are the variables that control this behavior? Research has shown that echolalia is controlled by a number of variables (Prizant & Duchan, 1981). However, for brevity, this chapter focuses on only one: poor comprehension.

To begin, it may be noted that young, normal children between 2–3 years of age display echolalia. Further, the behavior becomes less frequent as the children's language comprehension improves (Nakanishi & Owada, 1973). This observation suggests a relationship between level of comprehension and level of echolalia. Interestingly, the same correlation has been observed in the case of autistic children (Fay, 1969; Rutter, 1968).

This author and colleagues decided to test the notion that poor comprehension is a controlling variable for echolalia (Carr, Schreibman, & Lovaas, 1975).

Six children diagnosed as autistic or autistic-type were presented with a number of questions and commands. Through a series of pretests, Carr et al. (1975) were able to determine that the children had responses in their repertoires to certain questions (e.g., "What's your name?") and commands (e.g., "Clap your hands"). This author and colleagues guaranteed that certain other questions and commands would not be discriminative for particular responses by choosing a variety of nonsense stimuli to serve as the questions (e.g., "Bot ni ork?" and commands ("Mon dok ped"). In other words, the notion of verbal comprehension was made operational by defining it in terms of whether or not the questions and commands functioned as discriminative stimuli for specific responses. If the questions and commands were not discriminative, they were defined as incomprehensible. The results of this functional analysis were orderly and predictable. When questions and commands were presented that were comprehensible, the children gave specific, appropriate responses and typically did not echo. When the questions and commands were incomprehensible, the children echoed a great deal. Thus, the relationship between poor comprehension and echolalia was verified experimentally.

The significance of these findings can be made clearer by drawing a parallel between the results just described and the studies of the effects of easy versus difficult task demands noted previously. Specifically, incomprehensible questions and commands can be reconceptualized as difficult tasks. There are other data that support this notion. In the Carr et al. (1975) study, several children were preassessed to determine what types of questions and commands were difficult (i.e., frequently resulted in incorrect responses). A number of these questions ("What is a rose?") and commands ("Feel the cloth") were then presented to the children. Predictably, these language stimuli were routinely echoed. Since difficult tasks appear to evoke echolalia, the authors wondered whether the strategies already discussed for controlling behavior problems evoked by difficult tasks also applied here. This notion was pursued in a later research effort (Schreibman & Carr, 1978).

If echolalia is a response to difficult tasks, then it may be functioning as an escape response. That is, when a child keeps echoing a question, the teacher or parent eventually gives up and stops asking (i.e., the aversive stimulus is withdrawn). If this conceptualization has merit, then, keeping in mind the role of poor comprehension in echolalia, one may select an alternative response that serves the same function. A plausible alternative would be the statement, "I don't know." When normal children are confronted with difficult questions to which they have no response, they answer "I don't know," rather than echoing (e.g., "What is the capital of Nebraska?" Answer, "I don't know"). This reasoning would suggest that autistic children could be taught to answer "I don't know" to questions for which they had no answer (i.e., difficult questions).

When the child gives this answer, the teacher would presumably be cued to instruct (prompt) the correct answer. This result is functionally the same as removing the aversive stimulus. A difficult task is modified so that escape via echolalia is no longer necessary.

Schreibman and Carr (1978) implemented the strategy just described as follows. Children were taught to continue to give specific answers to questions for which they had an answer (e.g., "How are you?"—an easy question). However, they were taught to answer "I don't know" to questions that they were not able to answer (e.g., "Who is the president?"—a difficult question). A discrimination between these two types of questions, easy versus difficult, was taught in order to avoid a situation in which children learn to answer "I don't know" to all questions, even those for which this sentence would be an inappropriate answer. The data in Figure 3 represent two children's responses to the difficult questions. In pretraining (labeled "Pretest" in the figure), both children echoed all the what/how/who questions presented to them. In contrast, following training (labeled "Generalization Test" in the figure), each child showed increasingly frequent use of the sentence, "I don't know." Importantly, echolalia steadily decreased and was eliminated. Echolalia and saying "I don't know" were not physically incompatible responses. In training, for example, both responses would sometimes be given sequentially in answer to the same question. Since echolalia was not a target of intervention, but nonetheless changed, the decrease in this behavior represents a fourth example of response generalization. It could be said that the two response classes were functionally equivalent in that each expresses a lack of comprehension of verbal stimuli (questions). Alternatively, and less cognitively, one could say that each response functions to remove an aversive stimulus (difficult question) and, in this sense, one response is functionally equivalent to the other. This relationship is summarized in the fourth row of Table 1. Once more, response generalization appears to be mediated through the mechanism of functional equivalence.

EDUCATIONAL IMPLICATIONS

Thus far in this chapter, research has been described relative to four types of undesirable behaviors. Traditionally, undesirable behaviors, particularly stereotypy and severe behavior problems, have been dealt with by means of a variety of aversive or otherwise decelerative interventions. These interventions have been instituted on the assumption that before educational efforts can begin, undesirable behaviors must first be eliminated. The data presented here question this assumption. In every case, educational efforts preceded the changes observed in the inappropriate behaviors. Apparently, by focusing on response generalization possibilities, one can shift the emphasis from deceleration to ac-

WHAT/HOW/WHO QUESTIONS

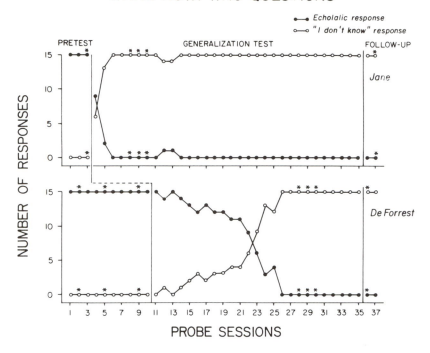

Figure 3. Number of echolalic responses given by each child to novel "what," "how," and "who" questions. Filled circles represent echolalic answers and open circles represent "I don't know" answers. Data collected by experimenters, who were naive to the purpose of the study, are indicated with asterisks. (Reprinted with permission from Schreibman, L., & Carr, E.G. [1978]. Elimination of echolalic responding to questions through the training of a generalized verbal response. *Journal of Applied Behavior Analysis, 11,* 459. Copyright 1978 by the Society for the Experimental Analysis of Behavior.)

celeration, from behavior management to skill building. Of course, it is true that there are instances of behavior problems that are so severe that deceleration is an immediate imperative (Carr & Lovaas, 1983). A child who head bangs to the point of bleeding or who bites others with such intensity that they require sutures may indeed require crisis management prior to educational intervention. However, the field has erred in generalizing from severe cases to all cases. The vast majority of autistic children do not regularly engage in life-threatening behavior. For them, the option of education first rather than management first may be a viable one. Even with severe cases, education ultimately becomes a necessity, since there is no other way of permanently replacing behavior problems. Perhaps the failure to achieve maintenance of treatment effects so often described in the literature may really represent a failure to educate rather than a need to develop ever more sophisticated aversive procedures (Evans & Meyer, 1985).

The study of response generalization has another implication, namely, that a child's behavior repertoire prior to intervention may be a valuable guidepost for selecting educational objectives. Traditionally, if one were teaching a child communication skills, one might attempt to superimpose on the child's existing repertoire a prepackaged language training program. Such efforts often fail. The failure quite often is related to motivational deficits. The child is said to be uninterested in the material being taught, or the child's newly acquired responses will not maintain unless arbitrary reinforcers (edibles) are made contingent on the language skills. One way of conceptualizing this problem is to make a distinction between form and function. The form, or topography of a behavior, may tell us little or nothing about the function or maintaining variables for the behavior. Thus, when a child says "juice" (a specific form), the word may function as a request for some juice or a description of the stimulus event itself, designed to evoke attention from an adult ("Yes, Jim, that is juice"). The ultimate task of an intervention agent is to assess what functions are currently in a child's repertoire and then to teach the child appropriate forms that serve those functions. Grafting arbitrarily selected forms (prepackaged programs) onto nonexistent functions is a prescription for failure, because the motivation necessary for maintenance is absent. In contrast, as noted before, a child's current repertoire can often provide a clear indication of what functions exist. Table 1 and the analyses that generated it can be an important step in deciding what forms to teach a child first. Thus, knowing that a particular form (screaming) serves an attention-seeking function should tell a teacher that a top educational priority must be to select a new form (e.g., verbal requesting) that serves the old function (attention-seeking); that is, functional equivalence must be programmed. The motivation (attention-seeking) for this new form is already present. What the child lacks is simply a socially appropriate form to serve the preexisting function. As has been seen repeatedly, selecting new forms (educational objectives) in this manner has the added advantage of eliminating old forms that are undesirable.

BEYOND FUNCTIONAL EQUIVALENCE: THE CONCEPT OF EFFICIENCY

As Favell and Reid (Chapter 8) stress, there are many variables that affect the generalization and maintenance of adaptive behavior. The concept of functional equivalence offers one relevant approach. An implicit issue involving functional equivalence, however, is how we can ensure that the adaptive member of two functionally equivalent behaviors will be the one that increases. Horner and Billingsley (Chapter 9) examine the problem within the context of a "competing behavior analysis." This author interfaces here with that analysis by emphasizing the important role of response efficiency.

Consider the example of severe behavior problems. As noted, when communication is strengthened, behavior problems decline, presumably because the two response classes involved are functionally equivalent. However, the mere fact of functional equivalence does not in itself explain the observed decline. Why, for example, does the child not retain both types of response? By doing so, the child would have two ways of getting attention, or escaping, as the case may be. To answer the question, one needs to go beyond the notion of functional equivalence. The author's working hypothesis, which is also the main focus of current research, is that functional equivalence is a necessary but not sufficient condition for some kinds of response generalization. For response generalization to occur, two response classes must not only be functionally equivalent, but one class must also be more efficient than the other.

Consider again the behavior problem example. Suppose an autistic boy screams whenever he successfully completes an independent work task. Further, it is empirically demonstrated that the screaming is typically followed by the teacher's talking to the child and asking him what he wants. This response is thus a useful way of getting attention. Why, then, would the boy cease his screaming over a period of time just because an adult teaches him to utter a phrase such as, "Look at what I've done," whenever he finishes a work assignment? The answer may lie in the concept of efficiency. Efficiency can be operationalized along at least two dimensions (Carr & Lindquist, 1987): reinforcement consistency and reinforcement delay. To illustrate, one might find that when the child screams, the teacher attends 50% of the time, but when the child uses the communicative phrase, the teacher attends 90% of the time. The communicative phrase and screaming may be functionally equivalent (i.e., they are both maintained by attention), but the former is more efficient than the latter with respect to the dimension of reinforcement consistency. Likewise, one might find that when the child screams, the teacher attends following a delay of 5–10 seconds, but when the child uses the communicative phrase, the teacher attends after a delay of 1–3 seconds. Again, the communicative phrase is more efficient than screaming, only this time with respect to the dimension of reinforcement delay. The author's preliminary data in this area suggest that the experimental analysis of efficiency may help throw light on the developmental issue of why one form of behavior eventually replaces another. Apparently, although the functions of behavior may remain constant over long periods, the forms serving those functions do not. Perhaps a more poetic way of expressing the same idea would be to suggest that while behavior forms may come and go, functions are forever.

CONCLUSION

Many mechanisms have been proposed to account for the phenomenon of response generalization (Voeltz & Evans, 1982). The present chapter has been an exercise in the analysis of one such mechanism: functional equivalence. The field is now wide open for a systematic analysis of other mechanisms. It is important to undertake this task. Understanding the various mechanisms involved will not only provide a meaningful treatment technology but may also constitute the basis for a theory of human behavior.

REFERENCES

Bandura, A. (1969). *Principles of behavior modification*. New York: Holt, Rinehart & Winston.

Bates, E., Camaioni, L., & Volterra, V. (1975). The acquisition of performatives prior to speech. *Merrill-Palmer Quarterly, 21*, 205–226.

Baumeister, A.A., & Forehand, R. (1972). Effects of contingent shock and verbal command on body rocking of retardates. *Journal of Clinical Psychology, 28*, 586–590.

Baumeister, A.A., & Forehand, R. (1973). Stereotyped acts. In N.R. Ellis (Ed.), *International review of research in mental retardation* (Vol. 6, pp. 55–96). New York: Academic Press.

Bell, S.M., & Ainsworth, M.D.S. (1972). Infant crying and maternal responsiveness. *Child Development, 43*, 1171–1190.

Berkson, G., & Davenport, R.K. (1962). Stereotyped movements of mental defectives. I. Initial survey. *American Journal of Mental Deficiency, 66*, 849–852.

Brown, P., & Elliott, R. (1965). Control of aggression in a nursery school class. *Journal of Experimental Child Psychology, 2*, 103–107.

Brownlee, J.R., & Bakeman, R. (1981). Hitting in toddler-peer interaction. *Child Development, 52*, 1076–1079.

Carr, E.G. (1977). The motivation of self-injurious behavior: A review of some hypotheses. *Psychological Bulletin, 84*, 800–816.

Carr, E.G., & Durand, V.M. (1985a). The social-communicative basis of severe behavior problems in children. In S. Reiss & R. Bootzin (Eds.), *Theoretical issues in behavior therapy* (pp. 219–254). New York: Academic Press.

Carr, E.G., & Durand, V.M. (1985b). Reducing behavior problems through functional communication training. *Journal of Applied Behavior Analysis, 18*, 111–126.

Carr, E.G., & Durand, V.M. (1987, November). See me, help me. *Psychology Today,* pp. 62–64.

Carr, E.G., & Lindquist, J.C. (1987). Generalization processes in language acquisition. In T.L. Layton (Ed.), *Language and treatment of autistic and developmentally disordered children* (pp. 129–153). Springfield, IL: Charles C Thomas.

Carr, E.G., & Lovaas, O.I. (1983). Contingent electric shock as a treatment for severe behavior problems. In S. Axelrod & J. Apsche (Eds.), *Punishment: Its effects on human behavior* (pp. 221–245). New York: Academic Press.

Carr, E.G., & McDowell, J.J. (1980). Social control of self-injurious behavior of organic etiology. *Behavior Therapy, 11*, 402–409.

Carr, E.G., & Newsom, C.D. (1985). Demand-related tantrums: Conceptualization and treatment. *Behavior Modification, 9*, 403–426.

Carr, E.G., Newsom, C.D., & Binkoff, J.A. (1976). Stimulus control of self-destructive behavior in a psychotic child. *Journal of Abnormal Child Psychology, 4*, 139–153.

Carr, E.G., Newsom, C.D., & Binkoff, J.A. (1980). Escape as a factor in the aggressive behavior of two retarded children. *Journal of Applied Behavior Analysis, 13*, 101–117.

Carr, E.G., Schreibman, L., & Lovaas, O.I. (1975). Control of echolalic speech in psychotic children. *Journal of Abnormal Child Psychology, 3*, 331–351.

Durand, V.M., & Carr, E.G. (1987). Social influences on "self-stimulatory" behavior: Analysis and treatment application. *Journal of Applied Behavior Analysis, 20*, 119–132.

Evans, I.M., & Meyer, L.H. (1985). *An educative approach to behavior problems: A practical decision model for interventions with severely handicapped learners.* Baltimore: Paul H. Brookes Publishing Co.

Fay, W.H. (1969). On the basis of autistic echolalia. *Journal of Communication Disorders, 2*, 38–47.

Forehand, R., & Baumeister, A.A. (1971). Rate of stereotyped body rocking of severe retardates as a function of frustration of goal-directed behavior. *Journal of Abnormal Psychology, 78*, 35–42.

Horner, R.H., & Budd, C.M. (1985). Acquisition of manual sign use: Collateral reduction of maladaptive behavior, and factors limiting generalization. *Education and Training of the Mentally Retarded, 20*, 39–47.

Kanner, L. (1943). Autistic disturbances of affective contact. *Nervous Child, 2*, 217–250.

Kemp, D.C., & Carr, E.G. (1986). *Preverbal requests: Joining the technologies of pragmatic language intervention and sufficient exemplar training.* Unpublished manuscript, State University of New York, Stony Brook.

Leung, E.H.L., & Rheingold, H.L. (1981). Development of pointing as a social gesture. *Developmental Psychology, 17*, 215–220.

Lovaas, O.I., Freitag, G., Gold, V.J., & Kassorla, I.C. (1965). Experimental studies in childhood schizophrenia: Analysis of self-destructive behavior. *Journal of Experimental Child Psychology, 2*, 67–84.

Mostofsky, D.I. (1965). *Stimulus generalization.* Stanford, CA: Stanford University Press.

Murphy, C.M. (1978). Pointing in the context of a shared activity. *Child Development, 49*, 371–380.

Nakanishi, Y., & Owada, K. (1973). Echoic utterances of children between the ages of one and three years. *Journal of Verbal Learning and Verbal Behavior, 12*, 658–665.

Prizant, B.M., & Duchan, J.F. (1981). The functions of immediate echolalia in autistic children. *Journal of Speech and Hearing Disorders, 46*, 241–249.

Rincover, A., Cook, R., Peoples, A., & Packard, D. (1979). Sensory extinction and sensory reinforcement principles for programming multiple adaptive behavior change. *Journal of Applied Behavior Analysis, 12*, 221–233.

Rutter, M. (1966). Behavioural and cognitive characteristics. In J.K. Wing (Ed.), *Early childhood autism* (pp. 51–81). London: Pergamon.

Rutter, M. (1968). Concepts of autism: A review of research. *Journal of Child Psychology and Psychiatry, 9*, 1–25.

Schreibman, L., & Carr, E.G. (1978). Elimination of echolalic responding to questions through the training of a generalized verbal response. *Journal of Applied Behavior Analysis, 11*, 453–463.

Shodell, M.J., & Reiter, H.H. (1968). Self-mutilative behavior in verbal and nonverbal schizophrenic children. *Archives of General Psychiatry, 19,* 453–455.

Stevenson, J., & Richman, N. (1978). Behavior, language, and development in three-year-old children. *Journal of Autism and Childhood Schizophrenia, 8,* 299–313.

Talkington, L.W., Hall, S., & Altman, R. (1971). Communication deficits and aggression in the mentally retarded. *American Journal of Mental Deficiency, 76,* 235–237.

Voeltz, L.M., & Evans, I.M. (1982). The assessment of behavioral interrelationships in child behavior therapy. *Behavioral Assessment, 4,* 131–165.

Wahler, R.G. (1967). Child-child interactions in free field settings: Some experimental analyses. *Journal of Experimental Child Psychology, 5,* 123–141.

Wellman, H.M., & Lempers, J.D. (1977). The naturalistic communicative abilities of two-year-olds. *Child Development, 48,* 1052–1057.

Williams, C.D. (1959). The elimination of tantrum behavior by extinction procedures. *Journal of Abnormal and Social Psychology, 59,* 269.

Wolery, M., Kirk, K., & Gast, D.L. (1985). Stereotypic behavior as a reinforcer: Effects and side effects. *Journal of Autism and Developmental Disorders, 15,* 149–161.

Index

A

Absenteeism, staff, controlling, 192
Adaptive behavior
  failure to generalize or maintain,
    reasons for, 198
  in unsupervised settings,
    promotion of, 121–122
Age mates, interaction of disabled
    children with, 81–82
Aggression
  communicative function, 226
  control, using delayed
    contingencies, 130–131
  escape function of, 227
  functionally equivalent
    replacement behaviors, 224
  functions of, 214–215, 226–227
  in autism, 13–14
  reinforcement, among peers, 144
  treatment, 171–172
  see also Problem behavior
*Assessment of Children's Language
  Comprehension* test, 27
Associated cues and effects, 79
  hypothesis of
    definition of, 89
    studies relevant to, 89–91
Association for the Advancement of
    Behavior Therapy (AABT),
    recommendations for
    behavioral interventions,
    179–180

Attentional processes, and
    motivation, 84
Attention-seeking behavior, 227
Audio recordings, mediational and
    conditioned stimulus
    functions of, 138
Autistic children/autism, 1, 2, 70
  conditional discrimination
    training, 26
  discriminative learning,
    reinforcers in, 89–90
  education
    motivational factors, 237
    and preexisting repertoire, 237
  excess behaviors
    control using delayed
      contingencies, 130
    reduction, 123
  failure to respond to
    environmental stimuli, 41
  generalization of behavior in, and
    stimulus input, 25
  generalization of treatment gains
    in, 21–22
  generalization tactics applied in,
    12–14
  improving motivation in, 46
  independent task responding of,
    with unpredictable
    contingencies, 126–127
  language acquisition in, 86–87
  learned helplessness hypothesis,
    45–46

R

S